D1602548

DYING INSIDE

Law, Meaning, and Violence

The scope of Law, Meaning, and Violence is defined by the wide-ranging scholarly debates signaled by each of the words in the title. Those debates have taken place among and between lawyers, anthropologists, political theorists, sociologists, and historians, as well as literary and cultural critics. This series is intended to recognize the importance of such ongoing conversations about law, meaning, and violence as well as to encourage and further them.

Series Editors: Martha Minow, Harvard Law School
Austin Sarat, Amherst College

DYING
INSIDE

The HIV/AIDS Ward
at Limestone Prison

BENJAMIN FLEURY-STEINER

WITH CARLA CROWDER

The University of Michigan Press

Ann Arbor

Copyright © by the University of Michigan 2008
All rights reserved
Published in the United States of America by
The University of Michigan Press
Manufactured in the United States of America
⊚ Printed on acid-free paper

2011   2010   2009   2008   4   3   2   1

A CIP catalog record for this book is available from the British Library.

Library of Congress Cataloging-in-Publication Data

Fleury-Steiner, Benjamin, 1970–
    Dying inside : the HIV/AIDS ward at Limestone prison / Benjamin
Fleury-Steiner with Carla Crowder.
        p.   cm. — (Law, meaning, and violence)
    Includes bibliographical references and index.
    ISBN-13: 978-0-472-11429-0 (cloth : alk. paper)
    ISBN-10: 0-472-11429-8 (cloth : alk. paper)
        1. Prisoners—Medical care—Alabama—Limestone.   2. Prisoners—
Health and hygiene—Alabama—Limestone.   3. AIDS (Disease)—United
States.   4. Prisons—Alabama—Limestone.   I. Crowder, Carla.   II. Title.
    HV8843.F58   2008
    365'.667—dc22   2008022948

*This book is dedicated to the memory
of a remarkable doctor and human
being,
Dr. Stephen Tabet
1962–2004*

*To all those who have needlessly
suffered and died in America's
numerous catastrophic penal
institutions*

CONTENTS

ACKNOWLEDGMENTS

I am indebted to Carla Crowder for her invaluable insight and her willingness to spend hours on the phone with someone who, until the year 2002, had never heard of Limestone prison. In addition to our conversations, Carla's insightful work as an investigative reporter for the *Birmingham News* enabled me to complete this book. Since leaving the newspaper for the rigors of law school, Carla was unable to participate in the writing of the manuscript. But after much insistence, she graciously allowed me to include her as coauthor. While I use "I" throughout the book, Carla's insights are present in everything I have written here. However, the views expressed in this book and any errors of fact or interpretation are absolutely my own.

This book would not have been possible without the remarkable support and assistance of the Southern Center for Human Rights (SCHR). SCHR staff members Tamara Serwer, Josh Lipman, and Lisa Zahren were incredibly generous with their time and willingness to share materials with me as the *Leatherwood* litigation unfolded. Lisa Kung, director of SCHR, provided invaluable clarifications toward the completion of the manuscript.

Other longtime prisoner rights activists also provided me with invaluable insights. Their willingness to spend hours sharing their stories was incredibly inspiring. The years of service they have dedicated to the difficult and often disturbing problems surrounding prisoner rights is, although they would never admit it, truly remarkable. I am therefore indebted to several of these amazing human beings, including Ellen Barry, Rachel Maddow, Jackie Walker, Cynthia Chandler, and the dozens of other activists and lawyers who appear pseudonymously in this book.

During the more than five years in which this project has developed, support from my colleagues in the Department of Sociology and Criminal Justice at the University of Delaware has been invaluable. I thank them all for taking the time to learn about a project that has quite literally consumed my attention for most of this new century. I also thank Rana Sachdev, Gina Julian, Matt Bacon, Brett Doe, and Kristian Wiles for transcribing interviews and offering reflections on various versions of the manuscript. I thank Jessica Hodge for collaborating with me in the first publication to utilize some of the data presented herein.

David Ermann, Aaron Kupchik, Laura-Beth Nielsen, and Michael Musheno read early drafts of the manuscript and provided invaluable comments and suggestions. Michael McCann invited me to present early versions of the project to his colleagues and students as part of a series sponsored by the University of Washington's Comparative Law and Society Studies Center, providing me with an opportunity to receive excellent feedback. During a conference entitled "Cause Lawyering and Social Movements" (held at the School of Law of the University of California, Los Angeles, on March 3, 2005), Rick Abel, Anna-Maria Marshall, Austin Sarat, Stuart Scheingold, Lynn Jones, and Steve Meili helped me refine my insights on the roles of lawyers and activists.

I thank Jim Reische and the University of Michigan Press for their patience and support. As I already mentioned, this project has been under development for well over five years, and without the press's willingness to let the project develop, none of what is presented here could have been possible. Moreover, the anonymous referees the press assigned to review the initial draft of the manuscript provided rich directions for revision and expansion. Their efforts have, in no small way, resulted in what I believe to be a far stronger book.

Most important, I thank my wife, Professor Ruth Fleury-Steiner, who over these many years has been nothing short of an angel. Her endless love and support have been extraordinary—especially as she was pregnant with our twin daughters during much of the final writing stages of this book. Ruth, I love you, Anna, Robin, and our three wonderful cats—Stanley, Misty, and Daphne.

INTRODUCTION

For nearly a decade, Dr. Stephen Tabet provided care to incarcerated HIV+ patients throughout the state of Washington. These prisoners nearly always suffered from multiple maladies, often a consequence of a long-neglected viral infection. In addition to HIV, several were infected with hepatitis C, a disease of the liver that is potentially lethal if left untreated. If one thing was clear to Tabet, it was that chronically ill prisoners typically had a myriad of serious health problems that demanded a comprehensive approach to their medical care—an approach he rarely saw in jails[1] and prisons in the United States or abroad. But Dr. Tabet was a committed and passionate warrior.

To put his experiences into proper perspective, Tabet had provided care for literally thousands of incarcerated patients with HIV and AIDS. Yet even this did not tire him out. When not on the inside treating prisoners, Dr. Tabet served as the director of the Northwest Correctional Medicine Education Program, where he taught other physicians and health care providers HIV medicine. Tabet also somehow found time to lecture on the topic in the United States and all over the world. Furthermore, he operated an electronic mail newsletter that provided advice free of charge to over 450 providers caring for incarcerated patients. But not even a seasoned, tireless veteran of prison medicine like Dr. Stephen Tabet could prepare for what he would learn about Limestone's notorious, segregated "AIDS colony." As an expert witness on behalf of the plaintiff class in the case of *Leatherwood v. Campbell,* Tabet's two visits to Limestone in February 2003 and February 2004 would reveal a situation confronting America's penal institutions that most could not have imagined would occur in this day and age.

Early Accounts of an "AIDS Colony"

Limestone prison is one of Alabama's newer facilities. Opening in 1984 in the northernmost part of the state, in a small town called Harvest, this rather drab facility was part of a broader plan to stem the tide of Alabama's long-term problems with prisoner overcrowding, a crisis brought to national attention by the ACLU since the early 1960s. Beginning in the early 1980s, several prisons were built in the northern part of the state with the specific objective of providing more cells. Hamilton prison, just southwest of Limestone, would serve to house Alabama's growing elderly prisoner population. Limestone would also play a unique role in the effort to stem the tide of overcrowding. Constructed in the early, often hysteria-filled years of the AIDS epidemic and wars on crime and drugs, the facility would serve as the sole institution for incarcerating all male prisoners in the state who were infected with the HIV virus.

An investigative report, "Inside an AIDS Colony," published in a 1991 issue of *U.S. News and World Report* by David Whitman,[2] is perhaps the most in-depth story ever published about HIV+ prisoners at Limestone. At this time, male HIV+ prisoners were segregated in Dorm 7, a facility known perversely to its occupants as "Thunderdorm"—a name adapted from a brutal arena depicted in the futuristic thriller *Mad Max: Beyond Thunderdome,* starring Mel Gibson and Tina Turner; in the film, prisoners were forced to fight to the death. Whitman wrote that in the context of Limestone prison, "Thunderdorm is a new kind of death row, one that houses every male prisoner in the state who carries the AIDS virus."[3]

Whitman and a photographer had remarkable access to the facility, conducted in-depth interviews with prisoners, and were able to question Limestone's warden at the time, J. D. White. Perhaps most strikingly, "Inside an AIDS Colony" presents disturbing photographs, including photos of its segregated trash dump and its morgue, as well as a haunting image of Adam Watts,[4] a prisoner who is shown chained in a shadowy lockup after having bitten a guard. From Whitman's account, we learn that Daniel Ryan was Limestone's first prisoner with HIV to be quarantined from the general population, in the early 1980s. The article begins by recounting in chilling detail what happened to Ryan on the fateful day.

> [W]hen the van pulled up to the gates of Limestone penitentiary in the fall of 1985, even Ryan failed to anticipate the reception that awaited him. The guards, normally scrupulous in searching a new prisoner, refused to touch him. Nurses outside his infirmary cell balked at even talking to him unless he first put on a surgical mask. When he showered, Ryan had to scrub the stall with pure bleach afterwards and mop his way back to his nearby cell, while armed guards in paper masks watched nervously. Ryan lived in isolation for five days, and then a doctor with a yellow mask came in and summarily announced: *"You have AIDS and are going to die from it."*[5]

Whitman's report features the plight of other prisoners newly quarantined in the months after Ryan's arrival, such as the gravely ill and terribly neglected Grady Thomas. The investigative reporter discovered that Limestone's nurses allowed Thomas to "lie in urine-stained sheets for hours."[6] Whitman also quite effectively solicited prisoners' emotionally jarring testimonies. Drawing on interviews with Ryan, other HIV+ prisoners, and Dorm 7's prison guards, "Inside an AIDS Colony" powerfully captures the climate of despair and hopelessness at the facility.

> The mental toll grew. Ryan and the other prisoners felt like spiders in a glass jar. Week after week, months stretching into years, there was no work or training . . . The lack of solitude and meaningful activity fed a loathing among inmates that extended not only to their guards and cellmates but to themselves . . . In time, [they] stopped answering their mail and taking showers and many abandoned their aspirations to learn a trade. "Every day," Officer Sam Mitchell recalls, "prisoners told me: 'I'm going to die. Why should I care what I do?'"[7]

Prior to Dr. Tabet's visit, there were two other noteworthy media profiles of Limestone's HIV+ prisoners. The first, a feature titled "HIV-Positive Inmates Face Prison within a Prison," appeared on a CNN Web site.[8] Similar to Whitman's article, the feature presents pictures of prisoners inside the unit's cramped quarters. In a chilling profile, one prisoner, Ralph Johnson, tells CNN reporter Aram Roston, "I accept death, personally I accept death." Also presented is a picture of a prisoner hugging a teddy bear, with the caption "Teddy Bears Provide Comfort for Some of the HIV-Positive Inmates." Another multipage feature, "Quarantined: Special Unit 16,"[9] appeared in Alabama's *Birmingham Post-Herald*. That story profiles a number of prisoners, including Arion Davis, who chillingly captured the atmosphere inside the unit at the time.

> There were so many people dying (in the HIV unit). It was kind of tough being around death. One day you're sick and the next day you're dead . . . For me I felt at one point, "When is my day going to come? Here I am serving a 17-year sentence and I'm waiting to die."[10]

The Present Study

As gripping as it was, one of the central limitations of the early news coverage of Limestone's HIV+ prisoners, as well as of the majority of popular discourse on prisons and prisoners in the United States more broadly (with the exception of some notable investigative reports that appear throughout this book),[11] is the failure of journalists to articulate the ongoing crisis as more than an anomalous case devoid of a broader social and political context.[12] Indeed, one of the great contributions of sociologists, political scientists, and prison historians has been to elucidate the ways in which jails and prisons reflect trends and conditions in the broader society of the time. This has been a growing area of interest over the last decade or so among sociologists, political scientists, and prison historians, especially those interested in the origins of mass incarceration in the United States.[13] But there are few ethnographic studies or intensive ground-level analyses of prisons and jails in the contemporary era of mass incarceration.[14]

The present study attempts to fill this void but is not ethnographic in the traditional sense.[15] Following the recent work of sociologist Eric Klinenberg in his case study of the Chicago heat wave of 1995, I begin with the assumption that "institutions have a tendency to reveal themselves when they are stressed and in crisis."[16] The Limestone case reveals a series of emerging and interrelated conditions, set against the backdrop of soaring penal populations and the loss of public accountability vis-à-vis the cutting and privatization of social services to the uninsured poor. These conditions include the incompatibility of health care and custodial discipline, the normalization of preventable suffering and death behind bars by overwhelmed medical personnel, and the pernicious effects of cost cutting as a central objective of penal bureaucracies in the nation at large. But before I detail how this case study will proceed, let me explain how the events that unfolded at Limestone are evidence of more than a "prison horror story."

The crisis of health care behind bars, especially among the most marginalized populations—the mass incarceration of poor, uninsured people with HIV/AIDS, hepatitis C, and other chronic and infectious diseases that can be dangerous if untreated—has given rise in the United States to what might best be called *catastrophic penal institutions*. This book documents the conditions that prisoners with HIV/AIDS were subjected to in one such institution in Harvest, Alabama—the only penal facility in the country that still enforces an open policy of segregating prisoners with HIV/AIDS from the general prison population. As conditions have worsened, the legal and other avenues for prisoners to challenge the grossly substandard medical care they are subjected to have narrowed. This has created a profound institutional crisis at Limestone and other jails and prisons nationwide.

Several factors explain why conditions have worsened. They include an overstretched prison system short on critical resources, the growing trend toward the privatization of medical care to save money, and the emphasis on security above all in the administration of penal institutions. Another factor is the strikingly similar way that politicians, public officials, and other commentators have framed the AIDS crisis and the war on drugs and crime. They have used a highly racialized rhetoric of hysteria to portray HIV/AIDS, drug abuse, and crime as problems that, if not properly quarantined and contained, threaten to invade and contaminate the wider public.

Chapter 1 of this book begins by reviewing sociological studies of prison that shed important light on how this institution must not be separated from broader societal changes. This material helps to reinforce the argument that "prison horror stories" appearing in the popular media tend to present a very limited view of why health care catastrophes take place behind bars in the United States today. The inquiry turns to how shifts in health care in the broader society cannot be separated from shifts in health care behind bars. My objective is to outline the institutional dynamics of catastrophic failure that occurred among Limestone prison's HIV+ prisoner population. I show that such an "anatomy of institutional failure" is not relegated to just penal institutions but also involves other institutions serving vulnerable populations, such as the elderly and disabled veterans. By exploring recent cases of neglect of the elderly and veterans, chapter 1 presents a clearer conception of what I call "captive conditions." The chapter concludes with a preliminary inquiry into how such conditions lead to serious breakdowns in the delivery of prison health care.

Chapter 2 picks up where chapter 1 leaves off. Specifically, in chapter 2, I explore in detail how both national and state-level shifts in penal policy and the courts shed light on the conditions that made institutional failure possible at such prisons as Limestone. I explore how the turn to mass imprisonment policies in the United States created a cost-cutting imperative at the state level. One of the most controversial means for cutting costs of soaring jail and prison populations has been the embrace of private prison health care providers by the majority of states.

Chapter 3 investigates the broader political shifts in the recent politics of law and order in the United States and the characteristics of those disproportionately affected by these policy changes—namely, poor, uninsured African Americans. In chapter 3, I ask why this population has been most effected by mass incarceration policies. Finally, chapter 3 explores how recent actions by the Congress have made it increasingly difficult for chronically ill prisoners to hold penal institutions accountable.

Chapter 4 builds on this line of inquiry by taking a closer look at the role that courts and lawyers have played in challenging the institutional context of prison medical failures. Specifically, I there show the crucially important—albeit flawed—role that courts have played in ensuring institutional accountability. However, a closer look at the passage of the Prisoner Litigation Reform Act of 1995 reveals that managing medical disasters and holding penal institutions accountable has become increasingly more difficult. The inquiry in chapter 4 focuses primarily on the detailed accounts of prisoner rights advocates currently working on behalf of HIV+ prisoners in the United States.

Chapter 5 demonstrates how broader shifts in penal and legal policy help to explain the specific circumstances surrounding the deaths of forty-three prisoners at Limestone in just over four years. The chapter focuses on the perspectives of the lawyers and investigators who represented the prisoner class, the way they developed their legal strategy, and the subsequent fairness hearing, *Leatherwood v. Campbell*. Taking federal magistrate John Ott's ruling in *Leatherwood* as a jumping-off point, chapter 6 explores in more detail Dr. Tabet's 2003 and 2004 reviews of the mortality rate of HIV+ prisoners. Specifically, my objective is to analyze what the circumstances surrounding prisoner deaths can teach us about the institutional failures that occurred inside Limestone's segregated Health Care Unit between 1999 and 2003.

The analysis of a failed system of health care at Limestone prison contributes a broader understanding of penal conditions in an increasingly punitive age. The analysis in this book will demonstrate how, at the institutional level of health care delivery, overcrowding, underfunding, and harsh living conditions have led to the veritable dehumanization of sizable populations confined in the jails and prisons all across the United States today. This finding should give pause to all those concerned with crime and punishment, irrespective of political ideology.

CHAPTER 1   Penal Health Care
in Contemporary
American Society

Sociologists of punishment have long recognized that inequalities in the broader society are mirrored in and through the prison population, beginning with such classic works as George Rusche and Otto Kirchheimer's treatise *Punishment and Social Structure* and Donald Clemmer's *The Prison Community*, a Depression-era case study of Illinois's maximum security prison at Menard.[1] As a staff member of Menard's Mental Health Office and a coach of the prison football team, Clemmer had unparalleled access to conduct both an extensive prisoner survey and a detailed field analysis of the institution. Clemmer's major discovery was that the prison's social hierarchy closely approximated the outside community. Specifically, he discovered that the prison contained three distinct classes: an upper class; a middle class; and a lower, "Hoosier" class. Alternatively, Gresham Sykes's *The Society of Captives*, a case study of New Jersey's maximum security prison (written at the height of the cold war, in the 1950s), focused more on the prison as its own self-contained social system. Ironically, of all sociologists to conduct the earliest investigations of penal institutions in the United States, Sykes most poignantly articulated the similarities between prison and the broader society.

In reality, of course, the prison wall is far more permeable than it appears, not in terms of escape . . . but in terms of the relationships between the prison social system and the larger society in which it rests. The prison is not an autonomous system of power; rather, it is an instrument of the state, shaped by its social environment, and we must keep this simple truth in mind if we are to understand the prison.[2]

Building on the insights of Clemmer and Sykes, one of the most sweeping sociological analyses of a prison is James Jacobs's study of the Illinois penitentiary at Stateville. Through archival analysis of fifty years of Stateville's institutional life and through rigorous observational analysis, Jacobs's book *Stateville* elucidates the rise and fall of various managerial approaches to prison governance that were shaped by and through broader societal developments. Most important for Jacobs was how Stateville had become shaped by the rise of "mass society"—that is, how the institution had been greatly influenced not only by officials but by social movements focused on creating a more socially inclusive, rights-based society.

The civil rights movement of the early 1960s served to politicize the prison minority's population which emerged as a solid majority by the 1960s. The trend toward mass society redefined the status and value of marginal groups in the polity. The demand by prisoners for fuller participation in the core culture was reinforced by the greater sensitivity of the elites to the moral worth of marginal citizens.[3]

One of the most compelling contributions of *Stateville* is Jacobs's discovery that a more activist judiciary was responsible for major changes at the institutional level of penal institutions. Setting forth a whole slew of new mandates designed to ensure minority prisoners' equal protection under law and to ensure the rights of prisoners to openly practice religion, Stateville underwent important changes, especially greater tolerance on the part of prison officials and the racial diversification of staff. Most of all, however, Jacobs discovered how the new legal mandates of mass society resulted in greater bureaucratization—in this case, a kind of symbolic deference on the part of Stateville's elites to new, legally mandated rules and regulations—as opposed to an idealistic view of prisons as places that put individual rights on par with the institution's overriding security imperatives. Indeed, Jacobs discovered that, on the whole, legal interventions resulted only in modest reforms into the 1970s.

> [T]ransformation was incompatible with the tenets of the authoritarian regime. It was also incompatible with the human relations model of management . . . The reforms mandated by the courts can only be implemented by well-run organizations . . . Whether rational administration and responsive grievance mechanisms will be sufficient to meet the press of inmate demands is a serious issue to be faced in the future.[4]

Understanding the authoritarian regime of the penal institution—what sociologist Erving Goffman, in the classic *Asylums,*[5] formulated as the "total institution"[6] (individuals living together twenty-four hours a day under a strict, depersonalizing climate of control)—is critical for understanding just how incompatible many of the court's mandates were rendered in the three decades after Jacobs's analysis of Stateville. Beginning especially in the 1980s (in the immediate years after *Stateville* was published), but accelerating in the 1990s, three trends occurred that greatly inhibited any movement toward a more humane and rehabilitative approach to incarceration: the near wholesale embrace of mass incarceration policies by a majority of American states,[7] the attendant massive overcrowding and the relative entrenchment of penal institutions as human warehouses, and a powerful backlash against prisoner rights by a far more conservative judiciary. Although I will discuss these crucial trends in subsequent chapters of this book (indeed, they will be fundamental to the presentation of the current study), it is important to note from the outset that, with notable exceptions in a few states that have resisted mass incarceration policies, these trends resulted in a reformulation of now severely overcrowded penal institutions.

Many of today's penal institutions resemble, perhaps more than ever before, the amoral bureaucracies brought most vividly to public attention in the wake of New York's infamous Attica prison riots of the late 1970s. The New York State Special Commission on Attica captured this situation and how it pertained specifically to deficient medical care.

No examinations were given at sick call; there was not enough time and neither doctor felt it was necessary . . . The approach was very businesslike, very direct, and very authoritarian. The time and effort necessary to explain, to help provide insight, to gain acceptance, to achieve confidence, were absent.[8]

Despite some important gains made in the treatment of HIV+ prisoners in the courts and by contemporary prisoner activists, many of the institutional-level failures described by the New York State Special Commission on Attica remain a pervasive part of the delivery of medical services to prisoners in the United States today. Overcrowding and lack of adequate resources in most states has made it all but impossible for chronically ill prisoners to receive consistent and adequate care. Moreover, the quick, "businesslike" approach by prison doctors at Attica is also realized today by most penal systems' increasing failures to conduct adequate audits and to keep reliable medical records in order to implement adequate protocols of preventative care. The term *businesslike* has largely taken on a distorted meaning when describing penal health care in the United States today. With the concomitant explosion, beginning in the 1980s, of such dangerous and complex chronic illnesses as HIV/AIDS and hepatitis C, along with the continued pains of tuberculosis outbreaks behind bars, economically overwhelmed states and local municipalities have relied on inexpensive, for-profit health care providers to manage the dying on the cheap.

Health Care Crises Inside and Outside U.S. Penal Institutions

Mirroring the broader societal trend toward cost cutting as the primary imperative of managing the health of marginalized populations in the United States, chronically ill penal populations are, drawing on Clemmer's prescient insight, representative of a microcosm of the broader society. The trend toward profit-driven private sector appropriation of health care—a trend that expanded most dramatically in the Reagan years and whose legacy continues into the present—has led to broad public dissatisfaction with the U.S. health care system. In addition, a recent study found that "17.6 million Americans—one in six insured adults, largely from middle-class families and holding full-time jobs—have substantial problems paying their medical bills."[9] The study also found that those who were insured but in financial debt had health plans of far less quality. A growing majority of Americans are experiencing the negative effects of what sociologist Paul Starr, in the classic *The Social Transformation of American Medicine*, has called "zero-sum medical practice."[10] In the context of deepening class and racial inequalities in the United States, the pains of for-profit medicine have been most acutely felt by the nation's marginalized populations. In their important, multivolume *An American Health Dilemma*, leading public health experts W. Michael Byrd and Linda A. Clayton observe, "Intentionally or not, the appropriation of the health system by capitalist market and corporate forces posed a clear and present danger to economically disadvantaged populations such as African Americans."[11]

With exploding numbers of poor, uninsured African Americans being locked away in the last three decades, America's grossly overcrowded and underresourced penal institutions have been impacted in dramatic and dangerous ways. To be sure, in the wake of the AIDS epidemic, activist groups in poor communities and inside penal institutions have played vitally important roles in educating marginalized citizens about the virus and helping to improve the overall quality of care. But as sociologist Rachel Maddow observes in a compelling recent study of HIV activism in penal institutions in the United States and Britain, the widespread embrace of privatized prison and jail health care providers has made this work exceedingly difficult. A recent report from the National Institute of Justice counsels that saving money may very well be the overriding institutional imperative of jail and prison health care providers in the United States today.

> Because prisoners lack the ability to consume all but the least expensive health services without the consent of prison officials, prison administrators have at least the potential to regulate prisoners' use of services very tightly. The ability to accomplish this depends in large part on the prison administration's success in controlling physicians' clinical decisions.[12]

Going Beyond the "Prisoner Horror Story"

This study employs most closely what sociologist Michael Burawoy refers to as "the extended case method"[13] (see appendix A for a fuller account of methods). However, by contrast to traditional ethnography, this analysis takes as its basis of inquiry one incident that has already happened: the deaths of forty-three HIV+ prisoners at Limestone prison in Harvest, Alabama, over a five-year period (1999–2003). Instead of casting the analytical net as wide as many previous studies of penal institutions have, I here explore these events as a means to investigate the world of contemporary penal practices in the context of the growing crisis of health care behind bars.

HIV/AIDS at Limestone Prison, 1999–2003

Early investigative reports of HIV+ prisoners held at Limestone prison provided important insights into the experiences of individual prisoners and their captors. However, based on these reports, one cannot help but be left with a rather narrow impression of the situation as an isolated "prison horror story"; that is, one is left to believe that this extreme situation of mistreated prisoners was driven by evil doctors and callous prison officials, without any documentation of the broader circumstances surrounding incarceration policies and prison health care at the time. By comparison, the words of the prison doctor who informed Daniel Ryan, "You have AIDS and are going to die from it" (quoted in the introduction to the present study), while callous, were uttered during the early years of the AIDS epidemic in the United States, a time when such overtly hysterical responses to those infected with the virus were commonplace in every region of the country.[14] Moreover, in the early years of the epidemic, the mainstream media's use of a tragic and hopeless narrative that emphasized a desperate attempt to contain the virus was routinely employed in dozens of stories involving doctors outside the prison system and their patients.[15]

The two interrelated dimensions left out of early coverage of the Limestone situation were the concomitant explosion of jail and prison populations and the loss, in many American states, of public accountability of state social services (i.e., the move to for-profit service providers). Despite the media's failure to make this obviously important connection, the AIDS boom hit state penal institutions hard. A combination of extreme prison and jail overcrowding with soaring rates of HIV/AIDS set in motion a deadly chaos behind bars that was not relegated solely to Alabama.[16] Yet the national media's focus on the sensationalistic nightmare of Limestone's "Thunderdorm" obscured these developments, which were important for understanding the crisis as more than an isolated incident.

Beyond "Thunderdorm"

The first glimpse at a more complex picture of the health care catastrophe at Limestone prison is presented in investigative reports written by Adam Liptak of the *New York Times* and *Birmingham News* reporter Carla Crowder.[17] Both Liptak and Crowder framed their articles within the bigger picture of prison overcrowding and systemic problems associated with prison health care more broadly. One of the primary reasons for this is that journalists were given access to the report that Dr. Stephen Tabet prepared as a medical expert witness for the *Leatherwood* litigation. Two astonishingly detailed volumes of more than two hundred pages in length, Dr. Tabet's report provided journalists an open window into the treatment, living conditions, and details surrounding prisoner deaths.

Dr. Tabet reported staff shortages and the use of an outdoor pill line to distribute medications, forcing immune-suppressed prisoners to stand in the cold predawn air. Drawing on such details, recent journalistic accounts moved beyond earlier, more sensationalized coverage of an "AIDS colony." Moreover, one article, "Prison Medical Failures Seen in Suit," documents for the first time how cost cutting played a major role in explaining how the drive to be "tough on crime" resulted in a dramatically compromised system of medical care in Alabama's jails and prisons.[18]

Providing a painstakingly detailed analysis of all forty-three HIV/AIDS-related prisoner deaths at Limestone between 1999 and 2003, Dr. Tabet's report provided journalists with a remarkably rich source of information. Indeed, the report gave journalists an account of the deaths documented by a recognized international expert on prison medicine. In contrast to the overwhelming majority of court opinions that rely on brief descriptions of broken prison health care systems, detailed reports that include prisoner death summaries are rarely made available to the press. Typically, prisoner death records are literally locked away from public view. Indeed, in recent years, few other state prison systems have made information regarding prisoner deaths widely available to the public.[19] Dr. Tabet's report thus provided information—about health care and the treatment of the chronically ill behind bars—that had long been obscured from public view.

The report focused mainly on the two key sites of HIV+ prisoner deaths at Limestone prison: Dorm 16, where the HIV+ prisoners had been housed between 1999 and 2003; and the Health Care Unit (HCU), which consisted of both an inpatient and outpatient unit.[20] His physical examinations of prisoners who had been living in Dorm 16 at the time of his visit and his evaluation of the institution's health care facilities provided a compelling commentary on the magnitude of the problem. However, Dr. Tabet's mortality reviews of the deceased would prove most crucial for understanding how the crisis at Limestone represented something far more than an isolated prison horror story.

Deadly Conditions

It is important to briefly summarize the most crucial details contained in Dr. Tabet's report. The seriousness of the situation is conveyed on one of the report's opening pages: "The HIV positive inmates are segregated into an HIV Dorm (Dorm 16) which is severely crowded."[21] Specifically, there were 250 HIV+ prisoners crammed into Dorm 16, a building that was not equipped for a population of this size. Also grabbing Dr. Tabet's immediate attention was the facility itself: Dorm 16 was an old converted warehouse. Prisoners slept in beds lined up end to end and side by side. Not surprisingly, signs of severe overcrowding—HIV+ men tightly clustered together and stagnant water from clogged shower drains—were immediately apparent. But only upon closer inspection did Dr. Tabet notice that the facility's physical structure had become seriously compromised. Many of Dorm 16's windows were broken. The doors lacked proper insulation and let in drafts, especially at night. During his visit to the facility in February 2003, Dr. Tabet also learned from several of the prisoners that the dorm was infested with insects, spiders, and vermin.

In the days just prior to Dr. Tabet's visit, a practice occurred that is all too common to prisoner rights lawyers and investigators. Literally within days of his visit, Alabama's Department of Corrections ordered very superficial repairs to the facility. In an attempt to mask Dorm 16's far more serious problems, prisoners and prison staff had given some of the outside walls a noticeably fresh coat of paint. It was also apparent that a few of the window screens had been recently replaced. In an attempt to cover the serious pest problem, the facility had likely been fumigated in preparation for Dr. Tabet's arrival. But dried rat excrement, evidence of Dorm 16's long-standing vermin problem, could not, as the report makes clear, be covered completely.

Once Dr. Tabet began to examine a few of the men living in the facility at the time of his visit, the catastrophic problems became all too evident. Numerous patients had evidence of severe skin infections, including pus-filled boils. The physical examinations of several of the men confirmed what was suspected all along by lawyers from the Southern Center for Human Rights: overcrowding and the probable influx of stinging and biting insects resulted in a staph infection that spread across the entire population of HIV+ prisoners. Indeed, many of the men Dr. Tabet examined had noticeable scarring from recently popped boils.

Dr. Tabet was also permitted to spend a considerable amount of time observing Dorm 16's outdoor pill line.

Patients at the Limestone Correctional Facility are administered medications at 3 a.m., 10 a.m., and 3 p.m. The patients are made to wait outside for their medications, often in very severe weather conditions.[22]

It became clear that this method for providing the dangerously ill their medications took far too long, especially for the weakest patients. Many of these prisoners were simply too sick to get out of bed. For those who could stand in line and receive their medication, another serious problem became evident to Dr. Tabet: all of the medications dispensed by medical personnel were placed in cups on the building's very dirty and decrepit windowsill, conditions ripe for contamination.

The layout of the segregated HIV prison facilities revealed other serious problems. Most obviously, Dr. Tabet was disturbed by the sheer distance from Dorm 16 to the segregated HCU. Walking the path himself, Dr. Tabet discovered that it took a full 20–30 minutes, an obviously ominous situation when one considers the heightened likelihood of medical emergency among such a gravely ill population. Once inside, the outpatient unit was a cramped—indeed, claustrophobic—facility. The physician and physician assistants were forced to share examination rooms. In such cramped conditions, it was impossible to even remotely ensure patient privacy or to provide proper care.

Dr. Tabet's visit to the inpatient unit revealed additional dire problems. For one, he learned from patients that the facility's emergency call buttons had long been inoperable but were repaired in anticipation of his court-ordered visit: "The inpatients are often too sick to leave their beds and find a nurse, and must use some sort of remote call device that is within reach of their beds."[23] A compounding problem in the inpatient unit was the use of prisoner "runners." Specifically, many of the prisoners became de facto nurses put in charge of the administration of nourishment to their often critically ill fellow prisoners. Obviously, Dr. Tabet found this practice in violation of all appropriate standards of health care for prisoners with HIV or AIDS. However, given the dire circumstances, ex-prisoners who served as runners, such as Wilson Rogers (see chapter 6), did provide invaluable support for prisoners in the final weeks of their lives.

Competing Accounts of Prisoner Deaths

The most devastating critique of Limestone's treatment of HIV+ prisoners came in Dr. Tabet's subsequent mortality reviews. All forty-three reviews combine to produce a compelling account of a profoundly understaffed, often unqualified, and overwhelmed team of medical personnel resorting to desperate and often disturbing measures. The mortality reviews provide detailed analyses involving the science of HIV/AIDS and numerous related infections and evidence documenting why health care delivery did not meet acceptable standards of modern medicine. Each review ends with an "impressions" section, where Dr. Tabet makes his outrage clear to even those readers unfamiliar with the complexities of HIV/AIDS in U.S. prisons. In this section, Dr. Tabet often describes treatment preceding death as "appalling," "unacceptable," and "completely inappropriate."

By contrast, an interview conducted by *New York Times* journalist Adam Liptak with Dr. Colette Simon, Limestone's medical director at the time of the deaths, as well as a transcript of the Southern Center for Human Rights' deposition of Dr. Simon, reveals an alternative account.[24] Responding to Dr. Tabet's report, Simon describes medical staff as doing the best they can in a situation that she admits is very difficult. Dr. Simon challenges Dr. Tabet's assessment as indicative of systemwide failure and instead describes a desperate situation that required her to take each case on an individual basis. Challenging Dr. Tabet's assessment that the deaths were the fault of the medical staff alone, Dr. Simon's most pointed rebuttal is one of prisoners refusing to be treated. But most broadly, Dr. Simon's testimony reveals a story of a physician entirely too overwhelmed to even consider recommendations made in a particularly critical audit of the facility conducted by Jacqueline Moore and Associates on November 8, 2002 (discussed in more detail in chapter 5). In response to the question of whether or not she read the report, Dr. Simon admitted candidly, "I never review this type of document extensively. For some reason, I find myself always too busy doing patient care."[25] Let us turn to both doctors' accounts in more detail.

Dr. Tabet's Story of a Broken Health Care System

Dr. Tabet would not learn of the most egregious medical failures at Limestone until he was able to thoroughly analyze the medical records of the recently deceased. While prison officials provided him only with records of prisoner deaths that occurred over a period of five years (between 1999 and 2003), Dr. Tabet's analysis is a scathing critique of an entrenched system of failed health care delivery. In contrast to sociological analyses that seek to understand systemic breakdown emanating from causes that go beyond formal health care practices, Dr. Tabet's report is, not surprisingly, one of a medical expert assessing whether or not prison health care administrators met acceptable standards of care. In other words, Dr. Tabet does not ask questions about, for example, broader political mandates involving cuts in social spending, imprisonment policy, the spreading of a deviant culture among medical staff, and how catastrophic loss of life became normalized inside the HCU, to see how they shed light on why so many prisoners died in such a short period of time. This is not to suggest that Dr. Tabet's report is conveyed in purely technical terms, completely devoid of emotion. Many of Dr. Tabet's assessments provide a forceful critique of the systemic breakdown of health care services that led to substandard care and, in many instances, deaths that he determined were largely preventable.

> In almost all instances death was preceded by a failure to provide proper medical care or treatment. Consistently, patients died of preventable illnesses. Patients with serious diseases experienced serious delays in medical care or were not treated at all. Chronic care clinics are unheard of at Limestone. Life-threatening laboratory results were treated routinely instead of urgently. Other tests such as radiographs showing pneumonia were commonly not assessed until many days later. At least one patient had such severe pneumonia that he suffocated in front of the medical staff—despite the patient's requests for treatment, he was not sent to a hospital until his condition was irreversible. CPR is rarely attempted in any critically ill patient that I reviewed.[26]

According to Dr. Tabet, a fundamental indicator that deaths at Limestone could have been prevented was the health care provider's inadequate documentation of cause of death. Dr. Tabet described how the absence of detailed and consistent record keeping could lead to the onset of an indeed deadly institutional inertia. By not having a systematic strategy for detecting commonalities in the causes of prisoner's deaths, the medical staff could not institute any preventative measures (e.g., consistent monitoring of prisoner nutrition and muscle mass). Dr. Tabet found, astonishingly, that medical staff did not conduct a single internal or external mortality review. The failure to keep adequate records and to conduct systematic audits was, as will be discussed in detail in subsequent chapters in the present study, not uncommon among jail and prison health care providers in other states. One unregulated cause of death that Dr. Tabet immediately observed was a strikingly high incidence of Pneumocystis carinii pneumonia (PCP), a disease that can be eradicated by treating HIV+ patients with an antibiotic called Bactrim, an inexpensive drug that costs literally pennies per day. Once PCP spreads, however, the price of treatment—figuratively and literally—rises exponentially. According to Dr. Tabet, treatment was the exception, not the rule, at Limestone.

> Patients at Limestone are treated like they are nuisances . . . This leads to lapses in medical care, increases the potential for resistant forms of HIV, and results in further mistrust by the patients in the medical system.[27]

Dr. Tabet discovered how the failure to conduct death summaries resulted in the spreading of other deadly conditions. AIDS wasting, in particular, had become widespread among the deceased. The lack of detailed records on individual prisoners caused wasting, a condition largely eradicated since the early years of the AIDS epidemic,[28] to remain a major, often lethal health problem at Limestone. Indeed, in many instances, Dr. Tabet discovered that undernourished patients were left literally to waste away. The overwhelming majority was severely malnourished; most had not received adequate nutrition or vitamin supplementation. Dr. Tabet's overall assessment of the situation did not split hairs.

> The conditions at Limestone Prison are unsafe for both the incarcerated and for the staff. There is a sense of hopelessness and helplessness among the patients at Limestone—to a degree that I have not witnessed prior.[29]

A final problem Dr. Tabet observed involved the dangers of conflicting goals between prison officials and Limestone's medical staff. Specifically, he discovered that dire situations involving prisoners in need of emergent care were trumped by the warden's overriding security objectives. Specifically, before an HIV+ prisoner could be rushed to an outside hospital for care, Limestone's administration required that the prison facility be completely shut down. All prisoners were returned to their cells, and the guards were placed on alert. In the context of a prison with more than two thousand prisoners, this procedure often took a considerable amount of time. Dr. Tabet discovered that the time lost by shutdown in the case of medical emergencies was very likely a direct contributor to several prisoner deaths.

Dr. Simon's Story of "Patient Rights"

While not explicitly addressing the social and political forces underpinning the medical care crisis at Limestone, the account by medical director Dr. Colette Simon is animated by a sobering commonsense view of prison health clinics as very challenging places to practice medicine and keep comprehensive records.[30] Dr. Simon, like jail and prison officials responding to health care problems in other states,[31] does not explicitly deny that there were serious problems concerning the care of HIV+ prisoners at Limestone prison. Rather, for Dr. Simon, confronting health care problems behind bars is unavoidably difficult; that is, from her point of view, penal institutions are problematic environments for managing chronically ill populations. For Dr. Simon, prison health care providers can only do so much.[32]

Dr. Simon's interview in the *New York Times* is the most detailed account ever published in the media. While the Southern Center for Human Rights (SCHR) did not name Dr. Simon as a culpable party in the class action lawsuit, a deposition conducted by SCHR attorneys is also revealing. Despite the fact that the plaintiff class described Dr. Simon as well-qualified and competent to provide HIV/AIDS medical treatment, her story reveals a taken-for-granted view of prison health care as very much dependent on the consent of individual prisoners.[33] From Dr. Simon's interview, one gets the sense that overcrowding and the penal system's grossly skewed ratio of prisoners to medical staff creates an inescapably difficult environment for providing health care to individuals with serious medical problems.[34]

From all accounts, it is clear that Dr. Simon never acted with any rational intent to harm HIV+ prisoners. She had a long and distinguished record of treating HIV-infected patients in other challenging environments, including many years in the most impoverished sections of her native Haiti. In short, Dr. Simon was anything but a villain who could be directly blamed for the catastrophe. Instead, the institutional conditions produced an overriding amorality among medical staff, as the interview with Dr. Simon revealed: "'All they have to do is come when they are called,' she said of the prisoners . . . Dr. Simon said that she tried to reason with and cajole prisoners in an effort to get them to take their medicine, but acknowledged that she did not always succeed."[35] The challenge of obtaining patient consent with medications is clearly real, as will be discussed in subsequent sections of this book. But health care providers—often with assistance of informed prisoners—have long implemented systematic strategies for addressing noncompliance, such as consistent follow-up and education.[36] Dr. Simon never mentions if such strategies were employed at Limestone. Instead, by focusing on the "right" of individual prisoners to refuse treatment, her response reveals a tactic that sociologist Michel Richard describes, in a case study of neglected elderly residents in one New York nursing home, as "the right to rot."[37]

Observing that there was a widespread level of resident inactivity and thus a dangerously high occurrence of muscular atrophy among the elderly patients in the facility in his study, Richard describes a typical staff response very similar to Dr. Simon's justification for problems associated with substandard care of HIV+ prisoners at Limestone prison. One nurse explained to Richard, "If patients don't want to exercise, we can't *force* them to exercise."[38] Additionally, this nurse and others told Richard that exercise was trumped by the staff's overriding concern for "patient safety" and the need to have elderly residents restrained. Richard cogently explains:

> I was not arguing that patients should never be restrained, I was simply asking that they be given more opportunity for exercise so that those who were still ambulatory would not lose the ability to stand erect and walk. The catch is that according to the medical model (actually a pseudo-medical model) patients do not lose the ability to stand erect and ambulate because they are tied up all day, but because of the inevitable progress of the disease. Coupled with the ideology of ageism, "patient's rights" translates into the "right to rot."[39]

There may have been some validity to Dr. Simon's claim that prisoners were acting on their right not to receive treatment, but as Dr.

Tabet's report makes abundantly clear, the situation at Limestone was far more analogous to an extreme version of Richard's "right to rot" story. In fact, it was obvious to Dr. Tabet that dying inside the HCU became the accepted rule rather than the exception. Dr. Simon's discretion was clearly characterized by a constrained bureaucratic logic aimed at "satisficing"[40] rather than optimizing care for prisoners' serious health issues. Coupled with an implicit ideology of prisons as inherently "difficult places to practice medicine" and of HIV+ prisoners as "noncompliant," Dr. Simon's account points to the importance of studying the Limestone case for what it can teach us about America's increasingly catastrophic penal system.

The Anatomy of Institutional Failure

A central contention of this book is that the events that occurred at Limestone prison between 1999 and 2003 were more than an isolated prison horror story in the extreme. The circumstances that made possible this catastrophic loss of life behind bars represent a microcosm of a broader set of institutional conditions that are vital for understanding increasing problems concerning chronically ill prisoners in the contemporary United States as a whole (see appendix B for a detailed inventory of cases involving catastrophic penal institutions from states in all major regions of the United States). Such deadly failures to prevent needless suffering and death in the nation's jails and prisons are the function of institutional failures that are routinely minimized by penal and privatized prison health care bureaucrats.[41]

The numerous medical catastrophes that occur behind bars do not simply result from issues specific to jails and prisons. What happened at Limestone prison will be shown as far more analogous to what sociologist Diane Vaughan has observed in her study of the complex institutional failures leading up to the disaster of the space shuttle Challenger, an incident that she argues was driven by incompatible organizational imperatives.[42] Faulty decision making that leads to disasters involving organizations, such as NASA, cannot be seen in narrow terms, as the behavior of a few "bad guys," but must be seen in terms of how the "organization structure facilitates misconduct as a solution to blocked opportunities by creating structural secrecy [and by] providing difficult-to-monitor mechanisms for carrying out illegal acts that conceal rather than reveal."[43] One of the unique institutional features of a prison, of course, is that it is a uniquely secretive institution; that is, in contrast to NASA, contemporary penal institutions are literally hidden from public view or scrutiny.

To understand how institutional failures happen behind bars, one must explore matters that go beyond jail and prison walls. In subsequent chapters of this book, it will become clearer that the story of institutional failure at Limestone is a complex tale of state and institutional authority run amok, as opposed to mistakes of individual actors. In their recent analysis of institutional breakdown at Abu Ghraib prison, sociologists Susanne Monahan and Beth Quinn observe:

> Focusing on the organizational structure within which deviance occurs leads to a set of questions that move beyond "who is to blame?" When the broader environment consists of competing or conflicting norms, organizational leaders and managers respond with structural arrangements that simultaneously absorb those conflicts and become the context for deviance.[44]

This book will demonstrate that two interconnected forms of institutional deviance, brought about by broader political and social conditions, were operating inside Limestone's HCU. First, the failure to keep adequate records and to perform annual audits led to a complete lack of preventative care on the part of Limestone's medical care provider. Second, the breakdown in preventative care at Limestone reveals specific ways staff normalized prisoner suffering and deaths. A central contention of this book is that both of these forms of institutional deviance are, to obviously varying degrees (see the conclusion of this book for a discussion of the far more humane and functional system of prisoner health care in Rhode Island), likely to be widespread among jails and prisons across the United States (see appendix B).

Not Just Penal Institutions

To understand why catastrophic institutional failures occur behind bars, one's investigation must go beyond the daily operations of prison and jail heath care providers. One must look into areas involving the often conflicting imperatives of the contemporary politics of law and order, prisoner rights protections, and the subsequent institutional pressures that mass incarceration policies have placed on prisons and jail medical systems in the United States today. The present analysis will reveal that at the institutional level of prison health care operations, the growing number of medical disasters taking place in the nation's prison and jails cannot be viewed as separate from the processes that explain catastrophic failures in other captive institutions, including veterans' hospitals, mental asylums, and juvenile reform schools. These institutions have disturbing records of emphasizing the control and isolation of captive groups, often at the expense of humane treatment and care.

A former head of the Massachusetts Department of Youth Services, Jerome Miller, writing in his important book *Last One over the Wall: The Massachusetts Experiment in Closing Reform Schools,* explains:

> In bureaucracies with a captive clientele the pull is always away from the personal and toward the impersonal and alienating . . . The pursuit is less one of public safety than of convenience . . . [Most] humane administrators eventually retreat to bureaucratic roles, trying to find peace in mitigating destructiveness.[45]

Miller's account documents how, in strikingly similar fashion to adult penal health care, a convenience-centered approach to the administration of Massachusetts reform schools was characterized by an utter lack of effective record keeping or proactive approaches to treatment. Miller's phrase "mitigating destructiveness" refers to an institutional response to system breakdown only after such damning events have been leaked to the media. Such responses are typified by an attempt on the part of high-level administrators to frame the situation as an "isolated event" that is the responsibility of lower-level personnel, who, as the recent scandal at Abu Ghraib prison demonstrates, are typically blamed and sanctioned.[46]

The case of disabled combat veterans is also instructive. While disabled veterans may have, at least in the popular imagination, more social status than HIV+ prisoners, VA hospitals have a widespread history of providing improper and substandard health care and of forcing patients to live in deplorable conditions.[47] Despite the myth of the honored disabled veteran, government cost cutting has historically undermined the quality of veteran care, as a leading historian of disabled veterans, David Gerber, has recently observed.

> Understandably, mythologies, histories, and other types of war narratives have long recognized the singular problem of disabled combat veterans. Their lasting impairments caused this recognition, and so, too, have popular narratives that valorize veterans' sacrifices on behalf of states and peoples. Such praise has nonetheless often stood in stark contrast to the neglect disabled veterans have experienced when war ended, memories faded, and governments, worried about large expenditures, declined to invest adequate funds to assist them in reconstructing their lives.[48]

Consider the recent scandal involving disabled Iraq War veterans confined in Building 18 of the Walter Reed Army Medical Center. As a special medical unit for Iraq War veterans suffering from serious brain injuries, this facility became a textbook example of how senior political and military officials retreat to a strategy characterized by mitigating destructiveness. Describing the conditions at Building 18 from the vantage point of one soldier's room, *Washington Post* investigative reporters Dana Priest and Anne Hull present a chilling picture of long-standing institutional failure at Walter Reed.

> Behind the door of Army Spec. Jeremy Duncan's room, part of the wall is torn and hangs in the air, weighted down with black mold. When the wounded combat engineer stands in his shower and looks up, he can see the bathtub on the floor above through a rotted hole. The entire building, constructed between the world wars, often smells like greasy carry-out. Signs of neglect are everywhere: mouse droppings, belly-up cockroaches, stained carpets, cheap mattresses.[49]

Since the scandal was brought to public attention, high-level military officials in charge of Walter Reed's operations have resorted to responses clearly aimed at mitigating the destructiveness of the situation inside Walter Reed. In responding to the conditions inside Building 18, some official (non)answers went even as far as to talk about plasma TV sets and the facility's other "luxuries."[50]

In the context of such resource-poor institutions as Walter Reed and Limestone prison, the mistreatment of disabled combat veterans and prisoners is driven by an amoral, often dehumanizing bureaucratic culture. Although all institutions must rely to some degree on formal, impersonal procedures for organizing large and complex populations, disabled combat veterans captive to a single institution for their care are particularly vulnerable. In *Achilles in Vietnam: Combat Trauma and the Undoing of Character,* a narrative history of traumatized Vietnam veterans, Jonathan Shay powerfully observes:

> Categories and classifications play a large role in the institutions of mental health care for mental health care professionals . . . All too often the mode of listening deteriorates into intellectual sorting, with the professional grabbing the veterans' words from the air and sticking them in mental bins.[51]

Captive Conditions

Prison and jail authorities in the United States have the longest and most troubling penchant for mitigating the destructive environments of penal institutions. This approach has been most pronounced in the revelation of decades of unregulated prisoner rape, beatings, and untreated or maltreated mental and chronic physical illnesses. To be sure, some state jails and prisons have better care systems in place than others (see the conclusion of the present study). Indeed, a study by the public health research firm Abt Associates found that an overwhelming majority of state prisons had proper medicines available to prisoners with HIV/AIDS. Most tellingly, however, the study's author, Theodore Hammett, cautions, "Those numbers look good, but there's quite a bit of information showing that there are a number of problems with access."[52] Indeed, Frederick Altice, director of Yale University's HIV in Prisons Program, challenges the Abt study's failure to confront what he believes is the essential story the data tell: that HIV prisoners are routinely denied access to treatment.

> If a prison has just one patient on a protease inhibitor, they can say on those surveys, "Yes, we provide it" . . . States don't want to say they are not providing the community standard of care. They can't afford to, because it's mud on their face. The real question would be, "What percentage of inmates with HIV has access to protease inhibitors?"[53]

Alabama may be the only state that still maintains a formal policy of segregating all HIV-infected prisoners in the state, but prisons and jails all across the United States use segregation policies that often result in blocking prisoner access to medication and thus in unnecessary suffering and preventable deaths. For example, New York prisons use isolation cells to segregate prisoners with tuberculosis, a practice designed necessarily to stop contagion but sometimes leading to lack of care and neglect.[54] The practice of segregating prisoners has, moreover, become intensified in recent years with the rise of Supermax prisons, facilities that keep prisoners in isolation for dramatically extended periods of time.[55]

The nexus of maltreatment and segregation is elucidated perhaps most glaringly in the case of mentally ill prisoners. A recent report by Human Rights Watch (HRW) documents how many mentally ill prisoners in the United States are left to languish in cells that are segregated from the general population. Specifically, "in the absence of meaningful psychiatric services," the report documents, "the afflicted prisoner's condition tends to deteriorate even further, and the long-term prognosis worsens."[56] Especially germane to the present study is the report's revelation that many prisoners kept in isolation often suffer from other illnesses, including HIV/AIDS and hepatitis C. Mental illness is common among prisoners with these chronic illnesses, and penal institutions rarely have adequate programs for dual diagnosis.[57] Perhaps even more striking is the report's revelation about the routine dehumanization of seriously debilitated prisoners. Rather than providing adequate care to such individuals, increased punishment becomes a kind of perverse treatment.

An important line of inquiry in the present analysis focuses on how broader social, political, and institutional arrangements help to elucidate the kind of catastrophic care detailed in the HRW report. But the primary focus here is on the HIV/AIDS epidemic behind bars. The next chapter begins by arguing that Limestone does not represent a "Southern anomaly" but is an extreme example of a set of institutional conditions that precipitate catastrophe in state penal institutions all across the United States. Chapter 3 will explore such conditions in a broader social and political context.

CHAPTER 2
The Conflicting Imperatives of Mass Incarceration and Prisoner Health

It may be tempting to write off the Limestone case as a problem typical only to infamous penal institutions in the southern United States. Given the historical record of brutal, inhumane conditions in prisons and jails in this region of the country—perhaps most notably the deplorable treatment of prisoners incarcerated at Louisiana's notorious Angola prison or Mississippi's Parchman Farm, the latter an institution that historian David Oshinsky famously described as "worse than slavery"[1]—one might conclude that the number of preventable deaths occurring among Limestone's HIV-infected population represents a disturbing regional anomaly. However, writing about the University of Pennsylvania Law School's Health Law Project of the early 1970s, public health scholar Douglas McDonald observed that serious deficiencies in the treatment of sick prisoners has by no means been restricted to the American South.

> The Project identified a number of deficiencies in Pennsylvania's prisons. Newly committed prisoners were given only cursory medical examinations, with no provision for ongoing medical surveillance. Access to "sick call," the only point of entry to medical care, was often barred by guards

who lacked training in medical triage. Special diets were virtually nonexistent; diabetics were simply told to select their food from regular meals, without instruction or assistance.[2]

Most recently, one need only take a cursory look at cases concerning health care for chronically ill prisoners in states from every region in the United States to realize that the nation is littered with penal health care systems that often fail to provide even remotely adequate access to treatment.

- In 2000, the *Milwaukee Journal Sentinel* reported that "dozens of Wisconsin inmates have died under questionable circumstances during the last decade in a flawed Corrections health care system that keeps internal reviews of prison deaths secret."[3] If not for a lawsuit and the newspaper's subsequent investigation of every prisoner death in the state between 1994 and 2000, the scandal would have remained the system's dirty secret. The investigation revealed that grossly understaffed medical care teams rarely administered CPR on dying prisoners; that emergent care was often dangerously delayed, resulting in preventable deaths; and that medical evaluations were often "sloppily done" and frequently did not even list the cause of death.[4]
- An investigative report of health care in all thirty-three of Ohio's prisons, conducted by the *Columbus Dispatch,* revealed catastrophic failures to provide care. A review of thousands of pages of records from the Ohio Department of Corrections and of dozens of interviews with prison medical officials uncovered that dangerously ill prisoners were routinely abandoned "after waiting nearly an hour for ambulances" and that "prisoners with chest pains died of heart attacks within minutes of being seen and released from clinics."[5] Additionally, dangerously ill prisoners at Lima Correctional Facility routinely went five or more days without receiving their prescription medication. In the most extreme instance, the prison's pharmacy contractor, Prima Care, left the prison's pharmacy completely unstaffed for two weeks.
- A yearlong investigation of health care practices in California

prisons, conducted by the *San Francisco Chronicle,* revealed "hundreds of cases in which sick inmates received care that was incompetent, negligent or punitive." The *Chronicle* reported: "Some inmates declined into critical illness before they recovered. Some were permanently disabled."[6] For example, despite repeated pleas to the officials at California's Avenal State Prison, HIV-infected prisoner Bruce Rizotto was called a "crybaby" by guards and left to die of an untreated respiratory infection.[7]

- As of 2006, the state of health care in California's prisons was so poor that U.S. district court judge Thelton E. Henderson placed the state's system under federal receivership.[8] A recent account by a court-appointed medical monitor, Dr. Robert Sillen, attests not only to the lack of adequate service but, indeed, to the persistence of preventable deaths in California's jails and prisons: "I have run hospitals, clinics and public health facilities for the past 40 years, and medical care in California prisons is unlike anything I've ever seen. Inhumane is the nice term for the conditions . . . Needless deaths occur weekly in our prisons, either from lack of access to care, or worse, from access to it."[9]

- A 2006 investigative report of Michigan's substandard jail and prison health care, conducted by the *Detroit Free Press,* found that numerous prisoners with life-threatening diseases went without treatment, often abandoned by medical personnel to deteriorate in their cells.[10]

- A 2005 investigative report of health care in New York's jails and prisons, appropriately appearing under the heading "Harsh Medicine," found that the state's private health care provider, Prison Health Services, woefully lacked adequate services. Indeed, investigative reporters found "repeated instances of medical care that has been flawed and sometimes lethal."[11]

Reports from Alabama, Wisconsin, Ohio, California, Michigan, New York, and other states from every region of the United States (see appendix B) make clear one of the most important characteristics of catastrophic penal institutions: by focusing primarily on punishment, custody, and discipline, these institutions are far from meeting the goal of providing adequate care to seriously ill prisoners.

The Prisoner as a Depersonalized Unit

The physical structure and internal organization of captive institutions is, in many respects, at odds with a well-organized approach to the delivery of medical care and treatment. While sociologist Marianne Paget's analysis of medical work outside the jail and prison context convincingly demonstrates that all medical work is "error-ridden, inexact, and uncertain because it is practiced on the human body,"[12] the case of the human body in the context of jail and prison health is especially problematic and in need of further clarification, especially given the captive culture of such institutions, which openly depersonalizes the inhabitants. Sociologist Nancy Stoller, a leading researcher on penal health care, provides perhaps the most in-depth analysis. Based on decades of research in California's prison system, Stoller observes:

> [T]he architectural and regulatory construction of prison naturalizes the prisoner as a depersonalized unit, teaching both the staff and the prisoner that this hyper-management and loss of agency is normal within the walls of this total institution . . . In prison, the body is all that the prisoner has. She is a number, a body to be counted for the regime but she is also a person. Staff members and prisoners learn the system of rules and the limits of life within them. The learning is structured by the process of negotiating the material location of the prison, as it is experienced daily. Over time, each prison's culture comes to be seen as a "natural environment," within which health care services are situated.[13]

The prison's "natural environment" of aggressive discipline and custody deeply inhibits adequate access to health care. In the extreme, dying prisoners, such as Bruce Rizotto, are primarily seen not as patients in need of serious care but as "crybabies." From the perspective of the prison's captive organization, such obviously demeaning and dehumanizing labels are a normal part of custodial behavior: Bruce Rizotto is first a prisoner to be disciplined; his identity as a human being to be cared for comes in at a distant second.

But as will become clearer in chapter 6 and is in evidence in appendix B, the Rizotto case is not indicative of the more pervasive institutional failures that render penal institutions in the United States today as ever more at risk for medical catastrophe. While it is often the case that guards and other line workers not affiliated with running the bureaucracy from the top become convenient scapegoats or representative of a few "bad apples,"[14] there are indeed some guards who act in ways that are considered truly deviant from a penal institution's professional culture and who are rightfully terminated from their duties. One only need consider a number of scandals involving guards participating in unprovoked acts of violence against prisoners to understand that serious problems may emerge within the subculture of correctional officers.[15]

Important changes in public policy shed light on the growing number of medical catastrophes that are taking place in the nation's jails and prisons. It is a primary contention of this book that one must investigate this broader context in order to understand how policies have led to profound institutional failures in health care access and delivery, particularly in the case of prisoners with chronic illnesses. This conceptual framework thus expands on previous research on dehumanizing penal health care in the context of the custodial subculture of the prisoner as a depersonalized unit. In addition to Stoller's research, the important work of criminologist Michael S. Vaughn and colleagues sheds light on the deplorable, often illegal actions of jail health care workers.[16] Vaughn's research sheds light on an increasingly dehumanizing form of incarceration in the United States—indeed, what some criminologists, such as Todd Clear, call a "penal harm movement," where the "essence of the penal sanction is to harm."[17]

Of Dollars and Lives: Why Study Limestone?

The discipline-over-care regime that undermines the humane treatment of chronically ill prisoners in the United States today is by no means a new development. However, a recent explosion in the rate of people behind bars points to a particularly troubling present. According to the most recent report from the Bureau of Justice Statistics, incarceration rates in the United States hit a thirty-three-year high in 2005.[18] Nearly 2.2 million individuals currently fill the nation's jails and prisons. Between 2004 and 2005, an additional 58,500 people were locked up. These historic increases have occurred despite continued declines in the national crime rate. A report by the Washington-based Sentencing Project states, "An examination of the rise of imprisonment from 1992 to 2001 concluded that the *entire* increase was a result of changes in sentencing policy and practice."[19] Although some states have begun to question the efficacy of harsh sentencing policies, the data clearly indicates that America is likely to remain a "prison nation" for the foreseeable future.

What mass incarceration and the subsequent push to cut costs has meant for the delivery of medical care to chronically ill, HIV+ prisoners at Limestone prison will be presented in chapter 6. But it is first important to note that medical catastrophes have taken place in the nation's jails and prisons ever since Walnut Street Jail, the country's first penal institution, opened in Pennsylvania well over two centuries ago.[20] Thus the preventable deaths of HIV-infected prisoners that occurred at Alabama's Limestone prison are not a unique event when considered alongside a protracted history of U.S. prisons and jails ravaged by tuberculosis and other infectious disease outbreaks.[21] If such crises are not new, why should we focus on Limestone? A central contention of this book is that comparing old and new penal health disasters is a distraction from what the Limestone case teaches us about an increasingly troubling present and what it foretells about future medical catastrophes that are ever more likely to occur behind bars, especially among prisoners in the United States who have debilitating, life-threatening illnesses.

Over especially the past thirty years, the United States has adopted an unprecedented policy of mass incarceration that takes Alabama's open policy of segregating HIV+ prisoners—a policy that explicitly emphasizes the control and isolation of a so-called risky population—as the modus operandi for managing the care of chronically ill and mentally debilitated prisoners in many U.S. penal institutions. In his important book *Governing through Crime: How America's War on Crime Transformed American Democracy and Created a Culture of Fear,* Jonathan Simon observes:

> The distinctive new form and function of the prison today is a space of pure custody, a human warehouse or even a kind of social waste management facility . . . The waste management prison no longer works through broad efforts at shaping personalities and personal relations of inmates

but relies instead on specific behavioral objectives to be enforced over any degree of resistance . . . [T]he order constructed by the toxic-waste-dump prison increasingly relies on total segregation of the prisoners considered most threatening.[22]

Simon arrives at this important conclusion based on his prior research of the historical development of parole in California[23] and of Project Exile, a recent federally promoted approach to mass incarceration.[24] Simon contends that this dramatic shift in prison governance is a relatively recent phenomenon, but when one considers the administration of health care, the model of exile and waste management has a lengthy history (see chapter 4 for how a waste management approach to prison health is revealed in legal cases going back to the early 1960s). At the same time, the recent explosion in jail and prison populations and the more overriding emphasis on waste management over rehabilitation, documented by Simon, vivify just how dangerous penal institutions have become for chronically ill prisoners in recent decades. With an overriding de-emphasis on penal institutions as places for rehabilitation and treatment, it is not surprising that to be chronically ill in the contemporary waste management prison is to be doubly at risk of unnecessary neglect and harm.[25]

Unable to meet the demands of exploding incarcerated populations of disproportionately uninsured persons with hosts of untreated, potentially deadly conditions, federal and state officials interested in being "tough on crime" have increasingly turned to controversial for-profit health care providers. In the case of Limestone, broader shifts in Alabama's political economy of imprisonment—for example, the consequences of Alabama's Habitual Felony Offender Act, the HIV/AIDS crisis in the state (e.g., the failure of the state to adequately fund prevention and treatment programs), and the dramatic undercutting of prisoner rights protections (e.g., the Prisoner Litigation and Reform Act of 1995)—shed important light on how forty-three preventable deaths occurred inside Limestone's segregated HIV prison in little more than four years (from 1999 to 2003). The explosion of penal populations, moreover, places tremendous fiscal burdens on state jails and prisons and makes it increasingly difficult to provide adequate health care to those with serious illnesses. This problem is compounded by the fact that many states, if not most, have dramatically cut social spending that addresses the needs of the unemployed and uninsured, while they continue to enforce regressive tax systems that tax those in the lowest income brackets. This state of recent affairs all but forecloses the spending of public resources to meet the needs of the incarcerated. As discussed in detail in the next section of this chapter, a chief way that states have confronted the fiscal burdens of mass incarceration is to hire low-cost, for-profit companies to run their jail and prison health care systems.

An Emphasis on Cost Cutting

In the early 1970s, many states switched to private prison health contractors because they were ordered to do so by courts that found their current services unconstitutional. Douglas McDonald observes, "In state prisons, the common pattern was for a federal court to find the state to be providing inadequate health care, court orders to remedy substandard conditions were then issued, and the government turned to contractors to remedy deficiencies."[26] With the explosion of prison and jail populations today, the overriding reason more and more states have switched to private contractors is that they believe it saves money. Whether or not this logic is actually correct is another matter. Indeed, McDonald reports a widespread "lack of systematic attention to outcomes of health care services" in the nation's penal institutions.[27]

Although measures of health care outcomes are weakly developed, a disturbing picture of serious deficiencies in privatized medical care in the broader public is emerging. Approaching health care according to a market model has resulted in less access to specialized, more expensive care for all segments of the population and thus in greater health care inequality. Public health scholar Mark Schlesinger observes, "Long-standing differences in health care utilization and health outcomes related to socioeconomic status or race are likely to grow under market reforms, as will other less visible forms of inequality."[28] While it is claimed that this reduction of costs results in lower premiums and thus greater access to care, one of the biggest controversies surrounding privatized health care in the United States is the bureaucratic red tape it creates for doctors. In the worst-case and increasingly common scenario, physicians are blocked from providing care to "higher-risk" patients that the corporation knows will require greater financial expenditures.[29]

If privatized health care is problematic for chronically ill patients outside the penal context, it is not surprising that such care has been substandard for prisoners. Indeed, prisoners are disproportionately poor, are more likely to lack medical insurance, and thus suffer from more serious health problems than the majority of the general public. Moreover, if privatized care is substandard or the provider denies treatment altogether, prisoners are not provided any health care alternatives.[30] Prison health law scholar Ira Robbins recently concluded:

[The] emphasis on cutting costs has created a well-documented risk that medical decisions are being based on financial considerations that result in constitutionally inadequate treatment. The prevalence of problems associated with privatized correctional care is sufficient to put jail and prison officials on notice of the risk that managed care practices will result in constitutionally deficient medical care. Thus, when an inmate . . . is seriously harmed and can demonstrate that this harm was the result of inadequate treatment or staffing, or any other managed care practice that creates an unjustifiable risk that financial concerns are being given priority over medical considerations, a rebuttal presumption that a policy or custom of deliberate indifference exists is warranted.[31]

The agenda conflict between privatized penal health care providers and public health advocates who work in U.S. jails and prisons is evidenced in a recent study by sociologist and longtime prisoner rights activist Rachel Maddow. An interview Maddow conducted with Ken Fields, a spokesman for Correctional Medical Services (CMS), a large private health provider, reveals cost cutting as the overriding imperative of such organizations. "We offer cost-predictability," Fields claimed, adding that CMS "can more accurately predict the cost of health care, especially when the environment and the standards of care are changing."[32] By contrast, Maddow's interview with a leading public health expert and recognized authority on prison and jail health care, Dr. Robert Greifinger, the former medical director of New York State's prison system, challenges Fields's notion that CMS can provide corrections officials with more control over problematic health care issues. Greifinger argued: "What makes them think that if they can't control it themselves, that they can control the vendor? No one has effective contract monitoring."[33]

How do actual legal cases involving for-profit prison health care providers shed light on this obvious conflict of interest? As it pertains to Limestone, this question will be answered more fully in chapters 5 and 6. Here, it is important to explore a previous case involving a jail in Georgia. As one of the first HIV/AIDS class action lawsuits brought by the Southern Center for Human Rights (SCHR) and involving a private health care provider, the Fulton County Jail case provides important insights into how problematic health care issues pertain to prisoners with HIV. Most important, this case clearly demonstrates the heightened potential for a conflict of interests between cost cutting and quality of care.

The Fulton County Jail Case

For much of 2000, prior to her involvement in the Limestone case, SCHR lawyer Tamara Serwer plunged headfirst into an extremely thorny case involving the utter lack of adequate treatment for HIV+ prisoners at Georgia's Fulton County Jail. In terms of the facts, the case did not appear particularly unique. Like so many of SCHR's cases concerning prison conditions, the litigation involved yet one more penal institution that was a train wreck of maltreatment and neglect.

Early into her investigation, Serwer and Joshua Lipman, an SCHR intern who, as an attorney, would later play an important role in the Limestone case, discovered that the HIV specialist in the jail insisted that HIV+ prisoners did not need lifesaving protease inhibitors. The discovery of protease inhibitors several years prior heralded a monumental breakthrough in the treatment of HIV. Taken orally in pill form, protease inhibitors block the protease enzyme that HIV needs to make new, potentially lethal viruses. Blocking the spread of HIV means less suffering and longer, healthier lives for patients. As public health scholar Theodore Hammett has observed, early access to such medication was problematic.[34] Yet as late as 2000, protease inhibitors were still not available at Fulton County Jail, so HIV+ prisoners there went completely without.

In addition to this compete lack of proper medication, SCHR discovered—from prisoners inside this grossly overcrowded, trash-strewn facility—that the doctor was maliciously judgmental of many infected with the virus. Specifically, Fulton County Jail's physician (not indicative of Dr. Simon or the medical staff at Limestone) would literally bring out a Bible and browbeat all HIV+ prisoners perceived to be gay. Once such a degradation ritual came to an end, the doctor would often dismiss the prisoner without treatment.

In addition to horrendous conditions and incompetent medical staff, HIV+ prisoners at Fulton County Jail were condemned to de facto segregation. These prisoners were separated from the general population and incarcerated with prisoners not infected with HIV but suffering from other illnesses. To streamline health care delivery, the county's private health care provider, Correctional Health Solutions (CHS), had placed all prisoners needing multiple pill calls in the chronic care unit to live together. Yet being thrust together with other non-HIV+ prisoners was not, as Serwer would learn, a problem for Fulton County Jail's HIV+ prisoner population. To the contrary, the community of chronically ill prisoners served a positive emotional function. Marlon Lewis,[35] the remarkably well-spoken and intelligent prisoner who wrote the original complaint against Fulton County Jail, explained in an interview after his parole: "We could be more open about our illness, and we weren't worried about the person behind us in the pill line for medication looking over our shoulder worrying about whether or not the guy behind wants to beat the shit out of you because you're HIV+."[36]

Many of the men in the county facility knew each other from the street. A vast majority were incarcerated at Fulton County Jail for drug-related offenses. As in many penal institutions across the United States, a disproportionate majority of the men were poor, black, and had lacked health insurance prior to incarceration. Many also had minimal education and did not have a genuine understanding of their illness. Serwer and her colleagues from SCHR discovered that a remarkably supportive community had emerged among the men.

They were educating each other. You know, the more educated or more sort of well-read or sophisticated guys would really try to tell the other guys, "You know, you need to take your medication, and this is why. And if you don't get it, you have to complain, like that's not good enough, because if you don't take this kind of medication the way you're supposed to, you could die!" They were compelling each other to try to take care of themselves. A good number of the guys—I mean, we saw so many deaths in that early part of the lawsuit—were actually cared for by each other, changing their sheets or helping one of the terminal guys. I mean, the nurses didn't want to touch them.[37]

But the strong community of support that emerged among HIV+ prisoners at Fulton County Jail was far from enough. Like so many other cash-strapped jails, Fulton County Jail's reliance on cheap, for-profit health care providers spelled disaster for the institution's HIV+ population.

Serwer convinced representatives from CHS and Fulton County Jail officials to discuss the problems of inadequate care. When the negotiations began, Serwer expected both parties to immediately resist SCHR's proposals to dramatically improve the treatment of HIV+ prisoners. Instead, a conflict between CHS and the county's attorney arose.

> We figured that both CHS and the county would disagree with us. But CHS actually agreed that the prisoners need better care. However, the county lawyers would oppose it—they would overrule the medical provider. The county proposed to do another evaluation, but the medical provider would be whispering behind their backs, saying, "We should do it faster than that." And the county would respond by saying, "You said you could address this with the contract that has been signed." In other words, the county knows this is going to cost more money to make the improvements that CHS says it can now put in place. In fact, it got pretty heated at one point, with CHS shouting at the county, saying something to this effect: "You wanted us to save you money, and now you're in trouble. What do you want us to do about it?!" So the county leaves the room and returns with a proposal to CHS, and this goes round and round for awhile. It's just extremely disheartening, because we have seen this kind of thing over and over again. Fulton County is a big, big jail so you are talking about millions and millions of dollars going into this. But, I mean, we are talking about a situation where people's lives are at stake! But for the county, it's all about money.[38]

Remarkably, Serwer finally convinced Fulton County Jail to make the necessary improvements to its system of health care.[39] If not for her skill as a mediator, the prospects of forcing Fulton County Jail to improve via the courts would likely have been an enormous challenge. While I will discuss the changing legal landscape around prisoner rights litigation in the next chapter, it is here important to explore briefly why seeking punitive damages against CHS would not have been a wise option for Serwer. Indeed, the chance of prevailing over a for-profit prison or jail health care provider in civil litigation has become increasingly remote, as Elizabeth Alexander explains in her essay "Private Prisons and Health Care: The HMO from Hell."

> The constitutional standard to establish liability on the part of officials is quite high. Staff must be "deliberately indifferent" to a "serious medical need." To prove deliberate indifference, the prisoner must establish that the staff member knew of a substantial risk of significant harm; the fact that the staff member should have realized there was a risk is not enough.[40]

As chapter 6 will clearly demonstrate, medical staff at Limestone rarely realized how serious the risks to dangerously ill prisoners were. By failing to have adequate medical records and thus preventative plans in place, catastrophic failure was driven by what might best be called "institutional indifference." But before turning to these and other relevant matters, it is important to see the Fulton County Jail case from additional perspectives.

The Fulton County Jail case reveals obvious problems in a system that, in effect, put a price on prisoners' lives. However, it also shows the remarkable resolve of a group of prisoners. Even at the hands of an excessively punitive physician who relied on a perverse interpretation of the Bible as a rationale for denying care, the men stuck together and created their own community of care inside the prison, a theme that is relevant to the Limestone case that I explore in chapter 6.

The Fulton County Jail case points also to a broader line of inquiry that serves as important background for investigating matters relevant to jail and prison medical catastrophes more broadly. Why do disproportionately poor, uninsured African Americans—the majority of the HIV+ population at Fulton County Jail and in the nation's penal institutions as a whole—comprise the group most likely to be subjected to substandard health care in the nation's overflowing jails and prisons? To shed light on that question, it is first necessary to take a broader view. The next chapter does this in a series of steps. It begins by exploring several important shifts in America's political order over the last three decades. Once this important contextual information is laid out, I then turn more specifically to the invidious effects of the racial politics of crime and punishment, to the broader socioeconomic conditions that precipitate health care marginality and poverty, and to recent court reforms that make it increasingly difficult for chronically ill prisoners to challenge the deteriorating conditions of their confinement.

CHAPTER 3   The Conditions That Produce Catastrophic Penal Institutions

The most influential work that provided policymakers of the late twentieth century with a clear conception and rationale for a newly invigorated strategy of law and order was conservative political scientist James Q. Wilson's *Thinking about Crime*. According to Wilson, the only realistic policy response was for government to address crime in terms of a cost-benefit analysis that emphasized crime control and the rational choices of criminals. As Malcolm Feeley describes it, Wilson's work became the "bible of the new criminology" and "shaped thinking about crime prevention at every level, from the White House to local police chiefs."[1] While Wilson's ideas were obviously very influential, it is critical to note that what ultimately led to the funding of harsh sentencing policies—and thus, in large measure, to their implementation—was the larger economic program that fiscally conservative legislatures from across the United States had begun to implement in the decades before the publication of *Thinking about Crime*.

If Wilson's *Thinking about Crime* was the new "criminology bible," economist Milton Friedman's *Capitalism and Freedom* was the bible of the new economy. Friedman's central thesis was that government's mismanagement of the U.S. economy was the chief cause behind the

Great Depression of the 1930s. But Friedman was hardly antigovernment. In fact, he vigorously argued for a centralized bureaucracy that would manage all economic activity through private entities and free markets. Friedman's neoliberal approach viewed the free market as the only viable response to addressing a slew of societal ills, from education to poverty—problems that Friedman argued government was not well suited to address.

Especially since the Reagan era, when Friedman served as a primary economic advisor, the privatization of government services in the United States has been widespread.[2] Military defense had been privatized long before. Since the 1950s, the U.S. Department of Defense had increasingly begun to rely on for-profit defense firms and contractors, in what President Eisenhower famously described as the rise of a "military industrial complex."[3] But it was not until the 1980s that Friedman's neoliberal strategy would have its most felt impact on everything from education to welfare and health care.[4] At that time, America's new war on crime and its aggressive incarceration policies would result in widespread state deregulation and, subsequently, in contracts to private companies involved especially in jail and prison construction, prison laundry, catering, and numerous other services utilized within penal institutions.[5]

Ironically, Friedman himself was no advocate of mass incarceration policies. In 1972, he wrote a *Newsweek* editorial calling for the legalization of drugs, and twenty years later, he criticized harsh sentencing laws as counterproductive.[6] But in a perverse irony, Friedman's call for aggressive privatization has endured as a driving force for sustaining the incarceration boom in the wake of policies of especially punitive drug sentencing and ending welfare as we know it. Indeed, in the last three decades, government-funded programs for poor, racially aggrieved citizens have been aggressively turned over to for-profit companies.[7] In the decade since the initiation of the welfare reform policy ushered in by Clinton-era U.S. Treasury secretary and neoliberal zealot Robert Ruben, economic inequalities in the United States have deepened, and incarceration rates have continued to skyrocket. By contrast to Friedman's vision of improved social welfare driven by aggressive private markets, moral objectives of helping marginalized communities through privatization have largely been undercut by the bottom-line cost-cutting mentalities of the for-profit companies that the U.S. government has increasingly relied on for running many of its crucial, traditionally public functions.[8]

This chapter demonstrates how recent policies of law and order and of economics converged with a politics of racial hysteria in ways that produced overcrowded, underfunded, and thus dangerously dysfunctional penal institutions in the contemporary United States. First, the chapter explores important shifts in crime and economic policy in the last three decades. I argue that to understand the rise of catastrophic penal institutions in the United States, one must consider the rise of mass imprisonment and the spread of the so-called market panacea concurrently. Next, the chapter examines the important link between race and the hyperpunitive turn, in the context of the passage of sweepingly punitive mass imprisonment policies in the late 1980s and the overpolicing and subsequent making of HIV risk populations in America's most marginalized communities.

The inquiry then shifts to analysis of the factors that produce the broader conditions of marginality that overwhelm grossly overcrowded penal institutions, making them ever susceptible to a health care catastrophe. The focus here is on the recent history of the explosion of the number of Americans who lack health insurance and on the crises that ensue for the uninsured with HIV/AIDS. Next, I turn to why the cycle of marginality continues in the United States and yields populations most vulnerable to the nation's hyperpunitive mass incarceration policies. Specifically, I argue that deepening racial segregation and a growing lack of employment and educational opportunities, a dramatic erosion of the welfare safety net, and punitive tax policies are all important factors for understanding how the catastrophic penal system in the United States emerged and continues into the present. The chapter concludes with an exploration into how recent legal "reforms" make it extremely difficult for HIV-infected prisoners to challenge the conditions of their confinement.

The Dangerous Nexus of "Tough on Crime" Policy and Aggressive Privatization

The rise of the conservative "tough on crime" movement and the embrace of privatization and the "market panacea" must be made a more explicit part of any analysis of the recent punitive turn in American policies of law and order. We must consider the broader consequences of such shifts concurrently. The seminal insights, nearly seventy years ago, of sociologists George Rusche and Otto Kirchheimer, who historically situated the analysis of punishment trends in terms that go beyond the confines of criminal justice policy debates and traditional penology, are all the more important in the current era of unprecedented punitiveness and privatization. Despite criticisms of their *Punishment and Social Structure* as too focused on shifts in the labor market for understanding the rise of imprisonment as the state's central strategy for containing the poor,[9] an emphasis on recent changes in economic policy is especially prescient for elucidating the institutional conditions—what Rusche and Kirchheimer called the "specific manifestations" of punishment[10]—inside U.S. prisons and jails today. While it is clear that an understanding of cultural and political forces are central for understanding the rise of mass incarceration policies (as recent studies by, e.g., David Garland and Marie Gottschalk convincingly show),[11] one of the principal claims of this book is that shifts in economic policy remain key for understanding the particularly harsh treatment experienced by the disproportionately poor outside and inside U.S. jails and prisons today. In addition to the morally potent conservative politics of law and order that Malcolm Feeley rightly argues must be made more explicit if we are to understand the dramatic expansion of penal institutions in the contemporary United States,[12] one must attend to the economic policies that have aggressively transformed punishment practices.

Sociologists Bruce Western, Katherine Beckett, and Loïc Wacquant have gone the furthest in showing how the dismantling of the U.S. welfare state has led to broader shifts in the utility of punishment—what Wacquant has termed "neoliberal penality." Wacquant explains:

> *The invisible hand of the market and the iron fist of the state combine* and compliment each other to make the lower classes accept de-socialized wage labor and the social instability it brings in its wake. After a long eclipse, the prison returns to the frontline of institutions entrusted with maintaining social order.[13]

Beyond economic instability, mass incarceration policies have created a perverse stability in unemployment among America's most marginalized, racially aggrieved citizens. According to Western and Beckett, the contemporary penal system in the United States has itself become a destructive, wholly regressive labor market institution.

> High incarceration rates lower conventional unemployment statistics by hiding joblessness but create pressure for rising unemployment once inmates are released. Sustained low unemployment depends, in part, not just on a large stage intervention through incarceration but on a continuous increase in the magnitude of this intervention.[14]

Broader negative shifts in the labor market and rising unemployment rates, particularly among marginalized populations, have been driven in substantial measure by mass incarceration policies. In the context of decades of sustained unemployment and poverty, there has been a substantial increase in the privatization of essential services. This growing use of companies focused on the maximization of profits to, in effect, manage a population that threatens its market viability has resulted in dramatic holes in the nation's safety net. Political theorist Wendy Brown offers an especially concise explanation of what she observes as the rise of a kind of socially Darwinist ideology of "self-care" that has been engendered by the profits-over-humanity objective of these social service corporations, an insight that goes a long way in explaining the lived experiences of increasing numbers of citizens and prisoners in the United States today.

> [M]ore than simply facilitating the economy, the state itself must construct and construe itself in market terms, as well as develop policies that promulgate a political culture that figure citizens exhaustively as rational economic actors in every sphere of life. Familiar here are the many privatization and outsourcing schemes for welfare, education, prisons, the police, and the military, but this aspect of Neo-liberalism also entails a host of policies that figure and produce citizens as individual entrepreneurs and consumers whose moral autonomy is measured by their capacity for "self-care"—their ability to provide for their own needs and service their own ambitions, whether as welfare recipients, medical patients, con-

sumers of pharmaceuticals, university students, or workers in ephemeral occupations.[15]

Those who are unable to engage in "self-care"—such as the uninsured chronically ill—are thus cut loose to the violence of current health care inequality; that is, if one is unable to negotiate the new, hyperindividualistic economy, the result is substandard health care or none at all.

Although several state policymakers and recent studies of public opinion are beginning to demonstrate a "softening on crime" on the part of the general public or, at the very least, a greater willingness to question the efficacy of what criminologist Todd Clear accurately describes as the "penal harm movement,"[16] significant damage has already been done over the last several decades. Investigating what mass incarceration policies have meant for the incarcerated, their families, the broader community, and the nation as a whole has taken on obvious importance.[17] We must then look at the fallout of aggressive incarceration policies beyond the confines of debates on criminal justice policy. In an important recent collection on the "invisible punishments" of mass imprisonment, Marc Mauer and Meda Chesney-Lind observe:

> Imprisonment was once primarily a matter of concern for the individual prisoner, but the scale of incarceration today is such that its impact is far broader—first, on the growing number of family members affected financially and emotionally by the imprisonment of a loved one; beyond that, by the way incarceration is now experienced by entire communities in the form of broad-scale economic hardships, increased risk of fatal disease … And ultimately, a society in which mass imprisonment has become the norm is one in which questions of justice, fairness, and access to resources are being altered in ways hitherto unknown.[18]

In the next section of this chapter, I turn to the community most impacted by mass imprisonment in the United States: African Americans.

Of Racialized Hysteria and Containment

In *Punishment and Inequality in America,* perhaps the most extensive empirical analysis of the costs of mass imprisonment policies for African Americans to date, sociologist Bruce Western concludes:

[P]oor and minority men were much less involved in crime in 2000 than twenty years earlier . . . . [A]lthough disadvantaged men became much more law-abiding [over this period], their chances of going to prison rose to historically high levels.[19]

Mass incarceration is not the result of "tough on crime" politics alone. Instead, as Gottschalk explains, recent surges in the penal populations came about not as the result of national politicians "finally discovering the crime card" but, rather, because of "how they played it."

Once the South reached détente with the rest of the country over the racial divide in the postwar decades as Jim Crow came tumbling down, federal law enforcement capacity expanded. Opportunistic local politicians egged on federal officials to expand federal policing and punishment powers. The debate over law and order no longer hinged, as it had for so much American political development, on fundamental questions of state power.[20]

Yet in Alabama and other states, learning to play the crime card has resulted in the passage of extreme punitive policies.

Even in the post–Jim Crow era, race has continued to play a critical role for invigorating both the federal and state government's power to use mass incarceration policies.[21] It is thus not surprising that African Americans have bore by far the strongest brunt of these draconian policies. The disproportionate warehousing of African Americans in the United States has ushered in a new epoch in the history of U.S. race relations that some have called the "New Jim Crow."[22] As the following subsection of this chapter will demonstrate, how politicians play the crime card has, in many ways, much to do with how they play the race card.

Playing the Race-Crime Card

Perhaps not ironically, the late George Wallace, the infamous racial segregationist governor of Alabama, is one of the central ideological forefather's of America's contemporary war on crime and drugs and its more than three decades of mass incarceration policies. "Wallace-style" crime fighting—dubbed the crown jewel of the so-called Southern strategy employed by opportunistic conservative politicians since the Nixon era—has been a driving force behind mass incarceration policies in the United States ever since.[23] Ironically, the Southern strategy was adopted at the national level by a Nixon administration once committed to a public health response to drug treatment and health care in poor, disproportionately black communities.[24] Desperate to court a white middle class shaken by the tumultuous years of the civil rights movement, the Nixon administration played on the racialized fears of civil unrest in the black community by subsequently forsaking the public health model for an all-out punitive war on crime and drugs.[25] In their authoritative three-volume tome *An American Health Dilemma,* W. Michael Byrd and Linda A. Clayton, commenting on the broader shift in the decline of black health after the passage of the Civil Rights Act of 1964, observe:

> Black health status deteriorated relative to Whites after 1980, with African Americans continuing to suffer excess morbidity and mortality and having the highest death rates in 12 of the 15 leading causes of death. The Black population began losing longevity in the mid-1980s for the first time in the twentieth century.[26]

Scholarly works have documented in detail how recent anticrime and antidrug strategies rest on several important assumptions about the failure of the liberal welfare state. Some of the core assumptions are that dangerous black criminals repeatedly go free because of left-leaning activist judges; that such prisoners are beyond rehabilitation and cannot be released safely back into society; and that more frequent and severe sentences are the only effective way to address crime, because they will contain this dangerous class of offenders, who are responsible for most crimes.[27] Fewer analyses focus on how this "updated" Southern strategy is silent on broader socioeconomic issues, such as lack of employment and educational opportunities in poor, marginalized communities and long-standing inequities in health care and access to programs for rehabilitation of substance abusers.[28]

In the context of an often hysterical, media-driven "crisis" of illicit drugs and "invading" populations of color, one principle way politicians were able to play the "race-crime card"—resulting in a dramatic jump in the U.S. prison population in the late 1980s—was to rely on a racialized hysteria narrative. Such a narrative drew both on the media spectacle of deaths of high-profile athletes, such as Len Bias, and on images of poor, black communities engulfed in a crack epidemic.[29] The central plotline was that crack addiction, confined once only to urban ghettos, had now begun to spread to more "respectable," disproportionately white suburban spaces. The story of a patently incurable "ghetto" now at risk of infecting suburban communities was embodied in the rhetoric of Howell Heflin, the Democratic senator from Alabama who cosponsored the legislation supporting a hundred-to-one sentencing disparity between federal crack and cocaine cases.[30]

> There is a violent war being fought in America. For many years this war was fought by special agents in dark, stinking alleys—through garbage-strewn streets, and in the burned out, abandoned buildings of our large metropolitan areas. But now, the battleground has moved into middle-class neighborhoods, into glass skyscrapers, and even into school playgrounds. This war was once fought only in urban America, [now] there are daily skirmishes on country roads, on remote rural routes, and in the tree-lined streets of small towns and villages.[31]

To be sure, it was not simply white politicians who embraced the hundred-to-one disparity and other wildly punitive antidrug sentencing policies, such as Georgia's "two strikes and you're out" law.[32] Many African American politicians were involved and complicit in the explosion of mass incarceration policies during this period of unprecedented expansion of the penal system.[33] This observation is critical to understanding why the racial hysteria narrative was so potent: playing the "race-crime card" has to do much more with conflating blackness and dangerousness than with one's skin color alone.[34] The story of a spreading, infectious, black crack epidemic was ultimately the quintessential rationale for ushering in "tough" sentencing policies, such as the hundred-to-one disparity. Contrary to the motivations of many policymakers who supported the policy as a way of addressing the problem of crack addiction in "the dark stinking alleys" of America's cities, the hundred-to-one disparity became law because of an overriding racialized hysteria over the spreading of the epidemic to the disproportionately white middle classes.[35]

Racialized Hysteria and HIV/AIDS

In a disturbing coincidence, at virtually the same time in history, the racialized hysteria narrative also drove the HIV/AIDS panic. Consider a 1986 *New York Times* editorial—entitled "Crucial Steps in Combating the AIDS Epidemic"—by leading conservative pundit William F. Buckley. In this piece, Buckley advocated for the tattooing of those with AIDS "in the upper forearm to protect common-needle users, and on the buttocks, to prevent the victimization of other homosexuals."[36] In the same year that the hundred-to-one disparity was passed into law, William Buckley called for an "AIDS tattoo" in the absence of any proposal for improved health care and treatment. Such a reactionary approach to AIDS in America has been ideologically realized in the government's overriding approach to addressing the epidemic in the most at-risk communities. Indeed, as Charles Perrow and Mauro F. Guillen explain, the Reagan administration took an openly hostile approach to the AIDS problem, blocking legislation and funding.

> The Reagan administration was particularly beholden to the moral majority and thus particularly unenthusiastic about taking action. Conservative groups reportedly were successful in blocking educational programs and limiting counseling services; it is possible that they even blocked appropriations for research, education, and treatment programs.[37]

There was also very little leadership on the part of African American political and church leaders. In *The Boundaries of Blackness: AIDS and the Breakdown of Black Politics,* Cathy J. Cohen argues:

> [T]raditional black leaders and organizations often engaged in their own process of secondary marginalization, where dominant discourses which sought to stratify and distinguish between "worthy" and "unworthy" marginal group members were replicated and in some cases adjusted to similarly mark and divide the more vulnerable segments of African-American communities living with AIDS. Ministers, politicians, and others with limited access to dominant resources distinguished between "innocent victims" of AIDS and those whose "bad" behavior led to their infection . . . With time this interpretation and discourse would come to include

more tolerant portrayals of, for example, injection drug users, but even today remnants of such ideologies still significantly structure the response to AIDS in black communities.[38]

Lack of leadership and, especially, lack of adequate funding to confront the AIDS epidemic have had obviously negative consequences for racially aggrieved communities. Rather than challenge the problem in terms of inferior health care and education, the prevailing politics has been characterized by racialized hysteria and an emphasis on dangerousness. In fact, since especially the late 1980s, the threat of HIV and drug addiction spreading to the privileged classes has been one of the main ideological pillars supporting policies calling for mass containment of these so-called threatening populations. The consequences have been all too obvious: the erosion of civil liberties embodied in racial profiling and other zero-tolerance policies that drive the contemporary drug war, the failure to address long-standing inequity in employment and educational opportunities, and the denial of a long-standing lack of adequate health care in communities of color.

The passage of the hundred-to-one disparity legislation and the call for draconian responses to the HIV/AIDS epidemic in poor communities were likely not intentionally racist responses driven by a blatant desire on the part of policymakers to uphold white supremacy.[39] Instead, the hyperbolic responses were driven by a hysteria that resulted in an aggressive policy imperative of appearing "tough on crime," a rhetoric that focused on the targeting of poor, racially aggrieved Americans. In clarifying how this one-sided mass incarceration strategy came about, the words of Nobel Prize winner Amartya Sen are particularly instructive.

> The asymmetry of power can indeed generate a kind of quiet brutality . . . [T]he inequalities of power in general prevent the sharing of opportunities. They can devastate the lives of those who are far removed from the levers of control. Even their own lives are dominated by decisions taken by others.[40]

In the policy debates fueling the wars on drugs and crime, the voices of the most affected populations were seldom heard.

The voices of those most affected by decades of mass incarceration policies have been largely silenced, and the consequences for those with HIV and AIDS have clearly been negative.[41] According to a recent report from the Bureau of Justice Statistics—entitled "Medical Causes of Death in State Prisons, 2001–2004"—more than twice as many African Americans than whites die of AIDS behind bars each year,[42] a finding that not only implicates the failure of state prisons to provide adequate access or care to such prisoners but also points to the larger failure of policymakers in the United States to ensure quality health care in economically marginalized African American communities more broadly. Assurances of such care have largely failed in a country whose political leaders of the last three decades have embraced a health care system increasingly driven by the bottom-line orthodoxy of for-profit health care providers. Deborah Stone powerfully observes, "Race becomes a proxy for factors that make a patient detrimental to the bottom line: chronic illness, prior inadequate care, and no insurance or underinsurance."[43]

Why Are Poor Blacks "At Risk"?

Before turning more explicitly to the broader issues of mass incarceration, for-profit health care, and racial inequality, it is important to consider questions that are implicit in much of what I have written about race, punishment, and AIDS thus far. What makes poor blacks most "at risk" for HIV infection? Has poverty created an "underclass culture" where risky sexual behavior and intravenous drug use is more acceptable than in more privileged communities?

Eva Bertram and colleagues convincingly shed light on answers to these questions in their important book *Drug War Politics: The Price of Denial*. Their book makes a convincing case that racial and class differentials in infection rates cannot be seen as "simply a reflection of urban poverty in the United States" or as resulting purely from "government neglect, although grossly inadequate social policies have set the stage for current conditions."[44] Specifically, Bertram and her colleagues make a convincing case that aggressive law enforcement strategies employed in marginalized communities as part of the drug war have inadvertently heightened the risk for HIV infection, particularly for injection drug users. Cathy Lisa Schneider has recently made similar observations.

> Intense police surveillance, combined with laws against possession of drug paraphernalia, has made the possession of clean syringes in minority neighborhoods extremely risky. Fear of arrest compels injection drug users to rely on syringes borrowed at the moment of injection. Second, persistent police harassment has promoted the spread of underground shooting galleries.[45]

Empirical studies of injection drug use by public health scholars provide strong support for Schneider's argument. Numerous epidemiological studies find similar rates of injection drug use between racial groups, but much higher rates of HIV-infection among such users in poor, racially aggrieved communities.[46] The reason for this differential in infection rates is straightforward: higher rates can be directly attributed to a lack of access to clean needles, coupled with a higher incidence of drug arrests. The consequences, as public health researcher Dawn Day concludes in a recent study, are disturbing.

> The legal system, via the police, is more likely to confiscate the personal needles of blacks. Also, because black users know (correctly) that they are vulnerable to arrest, these users are likely to "voluntarily" get rid of their own clean needles to avoid arrest.[47]

Of Mass Incarceration, HIV/AIDS, and the Erosion of Public Accountability

The consequences of more aggressive law enforcement that leads to the increased use of dirty needles and thus to higher HIV infection rates in many poor, black communities do not end on the street. Members of these infected populations are disproportionately arrested for nonviolent drug crimes and forced to serve increasingly longer prison sentences. Let us begin by looking at Alabama in the context of other U.S. states.

According to a recent report from the Bureau of Justice Statistics,

Alabama has the sixth highest incarceration rate in the nation, behind only Texas, Mississippi, Oklahoma, Arkansas, and Georgia.[48] A recent report by Justice Policy Initiatives, released in October 2005 and titled "Alabama Prison Crisis,"[49] explains why the incarceration rate is high particularly among Alabama's disproportionately poor, black community. While African Americans make up only 26 percent of Alabama's population, they account for a full 60 percent of the current prison population. Part and parcel to these disparities has been the criminalizing of poor, racially aggrieved populations that have been under siege by zero-tolerance law enforcement practices that hyperfocus on open-air drug markets common in such communities.

Once convicted, drug offenders in Alabama are subjected to the state's punitive criminal justice system. Alabama's sentencing structure exposes nonviolent drug offenders and other low-level offenders to repressive mandatory sentencing laws, such as its Habitual Felony Offender Act (HFOA). Since the reforming of New York's infamously harsh Rockefeller sentencing laws,[50] HFOA is the nation's most extreme sentencing legislation. Its harshness is noted in the aforementioned report by Justice Policy Initiatives.

> Alabama's Habitual Felony Offender Act . . . exposes defendants to sentences that are up to *ten times* the sentences permitted for first-offenders. Under the law, an individual charged with stealing $3,000 who has one previous felony conviction faces the same harsh sentencing range, 10 to 99 years, whether the prior conviction was for marijuana possession or murder. In fact, prisoners sentenced as "habitual offenders" were *twice as likely* to be serving time for property offenses as person offenses.[51]

One of the most obvious consequences of the HFOA and other mass incarceration policies in Alabama has been the tremendous overcrowding in the state's jails and prisons. Throughout the 1990s, the total state prisoner population grew by a full 70 percent. To put that into proper perspective, there are almost twice as many prisoners as the penal institutions in Alabama were designed to hold.[52] Indeed, by late 2005, the Governor's Task Force on Prison Crowding concluded, "The state's aging and often dilapidated prisons cannot be expected to serve its correctional needs."[53] At the national level, a recent overview by David Rothman of the extent of current overcrowding in U.S. prisons tells an equally grim story: "On average, federal prisons are 46 percent over capacity and state prisons are 31 percent. Cells built for one inmate often hold two or even three."[54]

From One Prison to Another: Declining Health, Opportunity, and Support for the Uninsured Poor

Lacking Health Insurance

In terms of state expenditures, Alabama spends approximately $8,128 per prisoner, by far the least among U.S. states.[55] The vast majority of Alabama's offenders that are locked inside its grossly overcrowded prisons and jails come from communities that are poor, lack adequate health care, and are most at risk for HIV infection. The Division of HIV/AIDS Prevention and Control of the Bureau of Communicable Disease under the Alabama Department of Public Health reports: "The number of Black males diagnosed with HIV/AIDS who are age group 13–24 and age group 50+ has increased by 89% and 24% respectively, between 2001 and 2005."[56] In a word, the lack of effective education and treatment for HIV/AIDS in poor Alabama counties has been devastating. As Jacob Levenson reports in *The Secret Epidemic: The Story of AIDS and Black America,* despite numerous advances in AIDS treatment, marginalized HIV+ residents in Alabama continued to go without.

> Alabama's infected tended to die quickly and were either too poor, too ashamed, or too isolated to make much political noise about their condition . . . They had virtually no resources to care for themselves.[57]

As of 2001, the average AIDS patient in Alabama made roughly seven thousand dollars a year. Only a few had health insurance. As Levenson demonstrates, a deadly nexus of poverty, lack of political leadership, and AIDS in the African American community forced the overwhelmingly uninsured in Alabama to turn to Medicaid and the federal AIDS Drug Assistance Program. But Alabama's failure to contribute a single cent to the federal program until 2000 put a dramatically tight cap on assistance in the state. Levenson explains the situation.

The waiting list had peaked out earlier in the year at 430. Those patients were dependent on local agencies like MASS (Mobile AIDS Support Services) to find the medications. Most often that meant that social workers had to fill out monthly applications for compassionate care programs set up by pharmaceutical companies. In 2000, for instance, MASS had "begged" for $1.8 million worth of medications from the pharmaceutical industry to cover its clients. And there was talk that some agencies had to secretly give out drugs they'd illegally stockpiled from the medicine cabinets of the dead.[58]

It is critical to note that while Alabama may be extreme in its lack of support for federal health interventions to combat the HIV/AIDS crisis in the state, Medicaid covered only slightly more than half of all Americans whose family income was below 200 percent of the poverty line in 2003.[59] In terms of access to public assistance by the poor, one must consider the real institutional problems associated with addressing the problem. First, it has become increasingly commonplace that public clinics across the country have become overwhelmed by bulging populations of uninsured Americans, and protracted delays in the delivery of care are increasingly the rule. Second, cashed-strapped hospitals often, perhaps out of desperation, twist the meaning of "charity care." In their compelling book *Uninsured in America: Life and Death in the Land of Opportunity*, a study involving dozens of uninsured citizens from every region of the United States, Susan Starr Sered and Rushika Fernandopulle chillingly conclude:

> Public clinics typically are so overwhelmed that the wait for an appointment can be several months. Hospitals often fail to inform patients that charity programs exist, instead simply billing their uninsured patients and turning their accounts over to collection agencies. In fact, although the government requires not-for-profit hospitals to offer charity care, many hospitals avoid doing so by redefining the uncollectible debt as "charity care."[60]

In the context of access to health care in penal institutions, prisoners are excluded altogether from Medicare and Medicaid benefits. Several states have also employed policies to dissuade prisoners from using health services, including requiring prisoners to pay co-pays and _fees. Ironically, as Douglas McDonald argues, this policy may actually cost penal institutions more money.

> Prisoners may not request attention for conditions that could turn worse, which then require more expensive care. If the marginal savings generated by lower utilization rates are small, and if the rate of emergency room visits increases by even a small amount, co-payment policies could result in higher expenditures for prison health care services.[61]

Deepening Racial Segregation and a Growing Lack of Opportunity

At this point, some readers may ask, why can't the uninsured (disproportionately poor and nonwhite) pull themselves up by the bootstraps and adapt to the changing economic conditions in the United States? While the answer to this question has received tremendous attention by social scientists and would thus require an entire volume to adequately answer,[62] it is important to note how one factor has caused the growing loss of educational and employment opportunities in the nation's most marginalized communities. Since the 1960s and accelerating into the present, cities in every part of the United States have experienced dramatic white flight.[63]

Taking vital employment and educational opportunities with them, working and middle-class white citizens have fled America's cities in droves over the last four decades. Between 1975 and 1980, Birmingham, Alabama, for example, lost a net of twenty-seven thousand residents to suburbia, accounting for a loss of more than half of its white population. Of the whites who stayed in Birmingham, approximately 80 percent live in neighborhoods segregated by race.[64] In a city where, for most of its history, many blacks lived in communities just outside the city, white flight has caused a profound increase in Birmingham's impoverished black population. Indeed, as social geographer Bobby M. Wilson has argued, such flight, coupled with a lack of transportation to the suburbs, has resulted in the vanishing of even notoriously poor-paying, underbenefited jobs in urban Birmingham.

> The suburbs employ many low-wage clerical workers and minority workers to clean office complexes and provide domestic services, reversing the

normal suburb-to-city commuting pattern. As a result, the supply of clerical jobs has become increasingly scarce in the central city, which consists mainly of low-income minority workers who must then commute to their suburban jobs . . . The result is a center-periphery pattern of development, with the central city increasingly on the periphery and the suburbs representing the center of growth and development . . . Blacks, portrayed as peripheral because of their color, now reside increasingly on the periphery and work in peripheral jobs.[65]

In addition to contributing to Birmingham's growing black underclass, white flight has impacted school desegregation efforts. Commenting on the isolating effects on urban Birmingham's students of color, Wilson observes, "By 1980, whites made up 44 percent of the city population but only 25 percent of the school population."[66] The effects of what Jonathan Kozol calls "educational apartheid" in the United States has resulted in grossly underfunded, understaffed, broken schools. Kozol reports that dramatically fewer poor, nonwhite students are graduating from high school today: "In 48 percent of high schools in the nation's one hundred largest districts, which are those in which the highest concentrations of black and Hispanic students are enrolled, less than half the entering ninth-graders graduate in four years. Nationwide, from 1993 to 2002, the number of high schools graduating less than half their ninth-grade class in four years has increased by 75 percent."[67]

Lack of Social Spending, "Welfare Reform," and Taxing the Poor

Compounding the deepening problems of racial segregation and the growing black underclass in Alabama and in an increasing majority of U.S. states are the added burdens many states impose on the poor. Alabama, like a growing number of states, spends very little on social programs. With the passage of the Personal Responsibility and Work Reconciliation Act of 1991 and the institutionalizing of a new federal system for managing welfare—Temporary Assistance for Needy Families, passed in 1996—the system has become ever more characterized by what sociologists Kenneth Neubeck and Noel Cazenave term "welfare racism."

Welfare racism exists as a major force shaping contemporary public attitudes, policies, and practices . . . It serves three major social stratification and social control functions: (1) *social* prestige for the general white population; (2) *political* and career powers for its politicians and other elites; and (3) *economic* acquisition for the nation's economic elite in the form of a large and easily exploitable low-wage labor pool.[68]

In terms of the economic function of welfare racism, Mary Bryna Sanger's *The Welfare Marketplace: Privatization and Welfare Reform* demonstrates support for Neubeck and Cazenave's thesis and builds on it by highlighting the troubling role of privatization as a vital aspect of so-called welfare reform. Although there is some variation in the particular models of service delivery, many privatized welfare companies, in consonance with for-profit prison health care providers, are focused first and foremost on saving the state money. For both welfare and health care, the consequences have been similarly troubling: insufficient care and a failure to ensure institutional oversight have been on the rise. In her case study of for-profit welfare service providers in San Diego, Milwaukee, New York City, and Houston—all locations that use for-profit companies employing different models of service delivery to welfare clients—Sanger concluded:

Adequate accountability and contract monitoring functions require far greater human capital and expenditures than are typically expected or budgeted for. Valuable and worthy nonprofits are becoming more businesslike; some have even formed for-profit subsidiaries . . . For all the improvements in performance that they promise, they raise troubling questions about quality and accountability.[69]

In addition to so-called welfare reform and the waning political will to seriously address problems associated with poverty in the United States as a whole,[70] another penalty imposed on the poor in Alabama is driven by the state's draconian tax laws. In 1933, an amendment to the Alabama Constitution gave the state authority to create a tax on personal income and set a limit of 5 percent for the tax rate.[71] Despite obvious changes to the Alabama economy over at least the last seventy years, this constitutional amendment has endured. Not surprisingly, the consequences of this long-standing cost-cutting mandate have been devastating to the state's most marginalized citizens: Alabama's poorest residents, including those below the poverty line, are required to pay very high taxes. The Alabama tax system also provides the lowest deductions for children, and a 1965 amendment has resulted in special breaks for those in higher income brackets. Barbara Larson, the executive director of the organization Alabama Citizens for Constitutional Reform, argues:

> Nearly 90% of Alabama's tax revenue is earmarked. The national average for earmarked funds is 28%, and we are at 90%. When our legislature debates the general fund, the debate concerns only 10% of the fund . . . The state can't spend money where it is needed the most in the short term, and we can't benefit from well-planned spending in the long term.[72]

In short, earmarking tax revenues—a process that is influenced tremendously by powerful special interest groups in the state—has, for more than seven decades, run amok in Alabama, leaving a tax base that is obviously very restricted.

Do the poor pay higher taxes in other states? According to a recent report by the Institute on Taxation and Economic Policy (ITEP), the answer is strikingly yes. The poor and middle class are taxed considerably more than the wealthy in every U.S. state. Like Alabama, states representing every region of the United States have particularly regressive tax systems, including Washington, Florida, Tennessee, South Dakota, Texas, Illinois, Michigan, Pennsylvania, and Nevada. ITEP concludes:

> These ten states ask their poorest residents—those in the bottom 20 percent of the income scale—to pay up to *five and a half times* as great a share of their earnings in taxes as they ask the wealthy to pay.[73]

Doing Prison Health Care on the Cheap

In the context of the "fiscal punishments" that are imposed on Alabama's poorest citizens, the effects of soaring HIV+ populations in the state's penal institutions are an important backdrop for considering why the state hired cheap privatized prison health care providers to manage Limestone's HIV+ population. The pattern Alabama followed for addressing health care crises behind bars is analogous to that followed by many, if not most, penal institutions in the United States, as Rachel Maddow explains.

In the 1980s, with rising prison populations already straining state budgets, US prison health care costs started to rise at a faster rate than the rest of corrections costs . . . To prison officials beset by rising numbers of prisoners, stretched health care budgets, the high incidence of expensive illnesses including HIV/AIDS, and the ever-present threat of Eighth Amendment lawsuits, private prison health care providers offered convenient-sounding solutions to longstanding problems.[74]

The hiring of private health contractors in penal institutions is also linked to state and local politics more broadly. In Alabama, Governor Donald Siegelman's role is crucial for understanding what would eventually transpire between 1998 and 2001. But a corrosive politics of health care in penal institutions is not a phenomenon unique to Alabama. Consider a recent case in New Jersey. In a move to save taxpayers hundreds of thousands of dollars, Passaic County officials fired sixteen nurses at the local jail and replaced them with a privatized medical contractor, Correctional Health. This move later became the focus of a federal corruption probe that linked Passaic County's Republican Party chairman to paid members of the board overseeing the county's correctional medical services. Since taking over the jail's health care services, several preexisting problems involving the delivery of medical services have worsened, including the failure to properly administer medications. Maia Davis reports, "The company's nurses are jeopardizing inmates' health by dispensing prescription drugs either too infrequently or in dosages that are too low."[75]

Recent empirical research provides further evidence of the influence of both political ideology and economic concerns as significant predictors of state decisions to use privatized penal service providers. Political scientist Sean Nicholson-Crotty argues that to accurately analyze the decision to use privatized penal services, an inquiry must consider the process in two stages. First, "states have enacted enabling legislation authorizing privatization in order to establish a legal basis for contract awards and preclude any challenges claiming that such delegation is unlawful."[76] In the second stage of the corrections management privatization process, administrators solicit proposals from private firms. Drawing on numerous statistical sources, including empirical data on state political characteristics, economic data that provide information on state spending limits, totals of state correctional expenditures as made available in the *Statistical Abstract of the United States,* and the Bureau of Justice Assistance's statistics on private prison contracts between 1996 and 1998, Nicholson-Crotty investigated both the enabling legislation phase and the contract negotiation phase. This research yielded two important findings: more conservative states were significantly more likely to pass legislation allowing for the use of privatized prison services, and states with stricter spending restrictions and higher total expenditures on prisons are more likely to have an active contract with such companies. Summarizing the broader implications of these findings, Nicholson-Crotty concludes:

> [B]oth economic and political factors influence state-level decisions to contract . . . The ideological orientation of a state plays a significant role in those decisions, with conservative states being more amenable to privatization. Numerous scholars have suggested support for market solutions to public problems is most often associated with a conservative political orientation and the results from these analyses confirm that insight in the area of corrections . . . Similarly, the economic influences on privatization found in other areas of public service delivery also seem to influence the decision to contract for management of corrections facilities. Disproportionately large budgets for corrections and the presence of limitations on the ability to raise revenues for future public spending of corrections services both increase the likelihood that a state will look to private contractors for a solution.[77]

Beyond the broader political and economic context of privatization, the record of for-profit prison health care providers has been less than encouraging. Indeed, there is ample evidence from around the country that institutional failure tends to characterize many, if not most, state jail and prison systems of health care. Nevertheless, Congress has taken active measures to make it increasingly difficult for penal institutions to be held accountable.

"Repeat Players," "Tough on Crime" Policy, and the Gutting of Prisoner Rights Protections

The U.S. government's approach to prison health care is particularly troubling when one considers that chronically ill prisoners depend on the courts to hold accountable the systems of substandard health care to which they have increasingly been exposed. As will be seen in the next chapter in this book, the unique role courts have historically played in governing prison health care has been dramatically narrowed by the passage of recent federal legislation aimed specifically at undercutting this obviously vital role. Perhaps most noteworthy is the Prisoner Litigation Reform Act of 1995 (PLRA), a law that has made it increasingly difficult for prisoners to challenge the conditions of their confinement.

To understand how the PLRA was ushered into law, one must attend to the broader political climate of the time. In 1994, under the leadership of Senator Newt Gingrich and Representative Dick Armey, the Republican Party took control of Congress by promising a new "Contract with America." Having successfully met many of their "tough on crime" objectives through the passage of a host of punitive laws (with widespread support from the Democrats),[78] Republicans drew on their successful antilitigation, "tort reform" rhetoric,[79] targeting it at prisoner lawsuits that they described as "out of control."

In a remarkable empirical study, Margo Schlanger presents both a sophisticated quantitative analysis of prisoner litigation trends pre- and post-PLRA and dozens of interviews with a host of relevant actors, including prison administrators. Her study documents how the PLRA drew immediate support from state prison authorities. Schlanger's interviews demonstrate that prison officials were particularly concerned that excessive prisoner litigiousness had created a culture of "repeat players" looking to file suit over any issue they could cook up. Consider Schlanger's characterization of an interview she conducted with the former head of corrections in Utah (now a national consultant on jail and prison litigation issues).

> He encouraged his staff and lawyers "to be warriors"—that is, to fight all litigation tooth and nail. He is proud, he says, that "in Utah, we treated litigation like a blood sport—got rid of all the lawyers who were the least bit afraid and hired warriors."[80]

To test the pro-PLRA thesis that prisoner litigation was out of control, Schlanger drew on archival statistical data collected by the Administrative Office of the U.S. Courts. While there was clearly an increase in the number of prisoner lawsuits filed in the 1970s, the 1980s, and especially the early 1990s, Schlanger found that "annual increases in federal civil rights filings were primarily associated, in nearly every state, with the growing incarcerated population."[81] Beyond the actual filing of a complaint, however, is how the courts have historically managed prisoner rights cases. Schlanger's analysis of every federal prisoner case between 1987 and 1993 demonstrates, in sharp detail, the utter lack of seriousness given claims of prisoner abuses by the courts.

> The average inmate civil rights case took under an hour of judge time, from filing to disposition. Because relatively few inmate cases settle, and because a small number of cases (the court order cases) can take up a very large amount of time indeed, an average of less than an hour means that judges spent little time on the rest, even though most of these remaining cases were resolved by courts rather than the parties.[82]

What effect has the PLRA had on prison litigation trends since the mid-1990s? Schlanger's analysis reveals that between 1995 and 1997, there was a 33 percent decrease in the number of federal case filings. The passage of state-level PLRAs suggests similar trends in state courts.[83] The federal government's overriding cost-cutting imperative has been dramatic, with nearly $20 million less spent on prisoner rights filings since 1995. Most distressingly, sizable numbers of meritorious prisoner rights cases have been dismissed in light of the PLRA. In particular, the PLRA's administrative exhaustion requirement that forces prisoners to use notoriously slow and ineffective prison grievance procedures before they are allowed to file suit—a provision that will be of particular relevance to my analysis of the Limestone case in chapter 5—has, as Schlanger argues,"effected a major liability-reducing change in the legal standards," because "inmates who experience even grievous loss because of unconstitutional misbehavior by prison and jail authorities will nonetheless lose cases they once would have won, if they fail to comply with technicalities of administrative exhaustion."[84]

Of Peanut Butter and Imprisonment

How were politicians able to pass such an obviously damaging law? It is important to explore this question in some detail. First and foremost, conservative senators—many of whom were former prosecutors and state attorneys general long known for aggressively posturing against "activist liberal" judges whom they tarred as responsible for the so-called litigation crisis behind bars—focused their attack on dramatically undercutting prisoner law suits. As the PLRA's chief sponsor, Senator Robert Dole turned to unreliable statistics and sensationalized accounts of prisoner "hyperlitigiousness" to demonstrate the need for an extreme legal response.

> The number of lawsuits filed by inmates has grown astronomically—from 6,600 in 1975 to more than 39,000 in 1994. These suits can involve such grievances as insufficient storage locker space, a defective haircut by a prison barber, the failure of prison officials to invite a prisoner to a pizza party for a departing prison employee, and yes, being served chunky peanut butter instead of the creamy variety.[85]

In addition to the so-called peanut butter case, attorneys general from around the United States testified at the PLRA hearings of prisoners suing over the color of bath towels and over not having a salad bar in the prison cafeteria.[86]

In a turn that is perhaps unsurprising but that is interesting for what it demonstrates about the powerful institutional momentum that federal "tough on crime" imperatives had generated in Washington, the veracity of the prison litigation abuse cases used by Dole and colleagues to rationalize the passage of the PLRA have been subsequently cast into serious doubt. Chief Justice Jon Newman of the Second Circuit Court of Appeals conducted his own independent review of the infamous so-called peanut butter, bath towel, and salad bar cases.[87] In the so-called salad bar case, Justice Newman discovered that forty-three prisoners filed a class action lawsuit filled with numerous and serious prison deficiencies, including overcrowding, forced confinement of prisoners with contagious diseases, lack of proper ventilation, lack of sufficient food, and food contaminated by rodents. Newman noted that the case's reference to salad bars in reality had to do with the prison's failure to address basic nutritional needs: "The complaint concerned dangerously unhealthy prison conditions, not the lack of a salad bar."[88]

In the so-called bath towels case, Justice Newman discovered that the case was not brought because of prisoners' color preferences for towels. The suit, in fact, focused on a prisoner's claim that the prison had unfairly confiscated the towels and a jacket that his family had sent him. Indeed, this prisoner filed suit because he was disciplined by staff simply for receiving a package from his family.[89]

In the now infamous so-called chunky peanut butter case, the wrong kind of peanut butter was not the actual reason behind the lawsuit. The prisoner filed suit because he was incorrectly charged for two jars of peanut butter. "Unfortunately," reports Newman, "the authorities transferred the prisoner that night to another prison, and his prison account remained charged the $2.50 for the item that he ordered but never received."[90]

Lawmaking and America's Punitive Wave

An exploration of the *Congressional Record* sheds further light on policymakers' narrow approach to lawmaking.[91] For one thing, the debate over the PLRA demonstrates a total absence of analysis of the ongoing crisis of maltreatment of the chronically ill and mentally debilitated. This is particularly noteworthy because lawmakers could have easily accessed an imposing record of legal cases, writings by prison health scholars, and accounts of former prisoners.[92]

Without a single mention of numerous reports documenting the crisis of suffering and preventable deaths behind bars, Dole and colleagues, by silencing these critical voices, participated in what Amartya Sen (quoted earlier in this chapter) called the "quiet brutality" of reckless authoritarianism. Rather than organizing a balanced debate around a serious, sometimes life-threatening set of issues, policymakers decided to focus exclusively on limiting prisoner litigation. For example, another feature of the legislation places a devastating burden on prisoners with mental illness. Absent a prior showing of physical injury, those prisoners suffering from the psychic violence of often serious, untreated mental illness were, from Senator Dole's perspective, examples of prisoners "playing fun-and-games" with the law.[93] Despite the well-documented evidence of the horrors of inadequate care, one must, in the parlance of the PLRA, be "tough" by imposing nearly impossible burdens on lawyers and judges regularly confronted with actual cases of grievous prisoner neglect.

Nowhere in the *Congressional Record* do we learn about the horrifying conditions of prisoners packed like sardines into the nation's many decaying and unsanitary jails, institutions where deadly tuberculosis outbreaks occur too commonly to this day.[94] There is no mention of the innumerable injustices of for-profit prison health care.[95] Despite the fact that many such accounts are documented in widely available court transcripts and briefs, not a single word was included about how, at the time the PLRA was signed into law, HIV-related deaths in the nation's prisons were at frighteningly high levels, while access to medication had become exceedingly difficult for those dying inside.[96]

Additionally, the PLRA dramatically limits attorney court fees, thus forcing underfunded and understaffed prison law organizations to deny even the most meritorious cases. Prior to the PLRA, attorney fees were waived, making it relatively easy for claims to be pursued. With the new filing fee and the requirement that prisoners seek relief from notoriously slow prison grievance procedures, even the most disturbing cases can be forestalled.[97]

Why was an irrationally "tough on crime" politics at the core of the passage of the PLRA? Prison psychology and law scholar Craig Haney eloquently describes the time: "The punishment wave . . . hit with such force that it . . . ripped us from the ethical moorings that once held this punitive system in check, kept us from straying beyond the moral outer limits of state-inflicted pain, and ensured that the course we set as a society for our crime control policy was guided, among many other things, by some minimal humanitarian considerations."[98] Indeed, PLRA co-sponsor Dole's riding of the "punishment wave" during the presidential campaign of 1996 was made abundantly clear in his visit to the notorious "tent city" jails run in the Arizona desert by Maricopa County sheriff Joe Arpaio. After a tour of a jail located in a place where temperatures routinely eclipse one hundred degrees and whose prisoners are forced to endure much of it as the result of the institution's ineffective swamp coolers,[99] Dole, revealing a potent rhetoric of cost cutting combined with well-worn "tough on crime" themes, told reporters that "other cost-conscious American communities" might copy Arpaio's desert jail model.[100]

The struggle on behalf of the chronically ill behind bars is a crisis with a very lengthy and often unpleasant history. In fact, the history of prison activism and prisoner rights jurisprudence reveals how the seemingly endless struggles over adequate health care for prisoners has been quite central to the history of the movement as a whole. Beyond the seemingly willful ignorance to this history by Congress are the consequences of the PLRA for chronically ill prisoners. It has, as will be analyzed in the next chapter, exacerbated the crisis confronting HIV+ prisoners and their advocates from around the United States.

The next chapter turns to the struggles of activists fighting for the lives of HIV+ prisoners in post-PLRA America. The chapter provides an account of how health care has, from the very beginning of the contemporary prisoner rights movement, been at the center of modern prisoners' rights activism and litigation. This account will provide critical insight into the fundamental roles that courts, prisoner rights attorneys, and activists played and continue to play in confronting the HIV/AIDS epidemic inside America's penal institutions today.

CHAPTER 4   Courts, Legal Change, and Institutional Struggle

It is clear that the birth of the prisoner rights movement in the United States cannot be separated from the emergence of the civil rights movements of the late 1960s. For the first time, the myriad injustices behind bars were made transparent to the general public. In addition to the racist, violent, and unsanitary conditions of the nation's jails and prisons, civil rights lawyers and activists exposed the near absence of adequate health care and prenatal care for incarcerated mothers. In a time when few, if any, organizers were working with incarcerated women or girls, the work of imprisoned black women activists, such as Angela Davis and Assata Shakur, paved the way for a far more expansive movement of the 1970s. Early into that decade, grassroots organizations, such as Aid to Incarcerated Mothers, Prison Mothers and Their Children (Prison MATCH), and Legal Services for Prisoners with Children, began to emerge around the United States.

These organizations drew explicitly on a radical feminist ethos that highlighted, among other concerns, the inclusion of all members, including former and current prisoners. Very early on, the line between prison and the community was blurred in the work of these organizations. Indeed, ex-prisoners were hired as staff, served on directorial boards, started new programs in their own communities, and were active members in shaping the identity of these early prisoner rights organizations. Ellen Barry, founder of Legal Services for Prisoners with Children, explained:

> We were then and continue now to be very conscious about building a class of people who see themselves as part of an organizing structure. They are part of an effort to change the system, whether it is about medical care or it is about expanding alternatives to incarceration for pregnant women or whatever. The idea is that we are all conscious of each other and thus are responsible to each other.[1]

The Struggle in the Courts

The early—and, in many ways, contemporary—prisoner rights movement is often characterized by a strong skepticism of litigation as a reliable tool for redressing prisoner abuses. However, as the movement began to pick up momentum in the sixties, so did the support for prisoner rights in the courts. Specifically, the Warren Court's revolutionary steps to protect basic prisoner rights under the Constitution ensured prisoners the basic rights to use the prison law library, practice their religion, and have access to lawyers. In the late seventies and early eighties, this trend in the courts toward upholding stronger prisoner rights protections continued. In perhaps its most pronounced affirmation, the Supreme Court ruled in *Estelle v. Gamble* (1976) that when prison officials are deliberately indifferent to the serious medical needs of prisoners, they are acting unconstitutionally under the Eighth Amendment's right to be free from cruel and unusual punishment.

In *Estelle v. Gamble*, a Texas prisoner, J. W. Gamble, was denied adequate treatment for a severe back injury sustained while performing a prison work assignment. Still suffering from his injury, Gamble refused to go back to work and was subsequently placed in solitary confinement. While the Supreme Court did not rule in Gamble's favor, it did take the opportunity to clarify a new standard—"deliberate indifference"—for what constituted "cruel and unusual treatment" of prisoners.

An inmate must rely on prison authorities to treat his medical needs; if the authorities fail to do so, those needs will not be met. In the worst cases, such a failure may actually produce physical "torture or a lingering death," the evils of most immediate concern to the drafters of the Amendment. In less serious cases, denial of medical care may result in pain and suffering which no one suggests would serve any penological purpose. The infliction of such unnecessary suffering is inconsistent with contemporary standards of decency as manifested in modern legislation codifying the common law view that it is but just that the public be required to care for the prisoner, who cannot by reason of the deprivation of his liberty, care for himself. We therefore conclude that deliberate indifference to serious medical needs of prisoners constitutes the "unnecessary and wanton infliction of pain."[2]

In the decades since *Estelle,* the Supreme Court has dramatically narrowed the meaning of "deliberate indifference." Rather than holding penal institutions accountable for indifference to prisoner suffering and neglect, the Supreme Court has placed on plaintiffs the burden of showing that their captors deliberately intended to do harm. Prison law scholar Susan Herman explains:

> New requirements grafted onto the Eighth Amendment focused the Courts' inquiry not on what treatment a prisoner should have a right to expect during confinement, but on whether prison administrators had behaved culpably and deserved to be punished. Prison administrators who remained oblivious to an inmate's need for protection, or perhaps even well-intentioned wardens who lacked adequate funding to maintain clean and safe institutions, now had a new defense against inmates' claims for minimally adequate treatment.[3]

Prisoner Rights from Below

A closer look at prisoner rights litigation reveals a sobering picture of a judiciary that itself has become increasingly indifferent to serious and obvious problems within America's penal institutions. Legal scholars of prisoner rights have for many years described the difficulties in gauging the effects of prison reform.[4] To be sure, judges in seemingly countless numbers of cases have repeatedly ordered prison officials to improve their health care systems. To some extent, direct judicial action has resulted in positive outcomes, including the improved quality of prison medical staff and the adoption of national standards of care by some state institutions.[5] But beyond the managerial actions of judges—that is, authorizing prisoner rights from "above"—another struggle over prison conditions and especially prisoner health has taken place from "below," in the actions of prisoner activists and advocates working in the nation's penal institutions.

When considering the early years of the movement, civil rights lawyers and activists since the sixties have been involved in prison conditions cases in a number of significant ways. Margo Schlanger reports, "A number of the lawyers who represented plaintiffs in the core cases of the movement—school desegregation, voting rights, criminal defense of civil rights protestors, and the like—started doing prison litigation after, in a sense, 'following their clients into jail.'"[6] At the national level, the NAACP Legal Defense and Education Fund (LDF) was the first national group to wage a massive litigation campaign against prisons with deplorable conditions, including the racial segregation of prisoners at Mississippi's notorious Parchman Farm.[7]

Since the 1960s and lasting for nearly two decades, federal judge Frank Johnson Jr. and attorney Larry Yackle of the ACLU National Prison Project (NPP), aggressively tried to reform Alabama's glaringly cruel and unusual prison conditions and inept system of health care delivery. In a series of cases throughout the late sixties, the seventies, and the early eighties, Judge Johnson ordered the Alabama Department of Corrections to make a number of systematic reforms to address persistent problems of prisoner overcrowding and deplorable conditions of confinement, along with numerous other issues.[8] Writing nearly three decades prior to the *Leatherwood* litigation brought to court by the Southern Center of Human Rights, Judge Johnson would confront similar issues as the judge in the Limestone case and order medical officials at Alabama's Kilby Prison to make a number of reforms to its grossly deficient health care system, including its inhumane policy of segregating all prisoners with hepatitis.

No effort has been made to bring the Medical and Diagnostic Center at Kilby into compliance with the minimum Medicare standards as required by the Court. A lack of professionalism characterizes the administration of the prison hospital . . . Patients with different strains of hepatitis have been placed in the same ward at great risk to life. There is no hospital dietician and no medical records librarian. A laboratory technician has been serving as hospital administrator. These conditions amply reflect that the medical director has failed to comply with the order of the Court that he develop a program of continual evaluation of all facilities and all personnel. The delivery of medical care in the Alabama Prison System is not characterized by poor management, but by no management.[9]

Prisoner rights litigation picked up steam in the early 1970s, after the notorious Attica prison riots. In the years after Attica, the NPP kicked into high gear, aggressively challenging deplorable conditions in jails and prisons all over the United States. The NPP won a remarkable number of cases, convincing judges to become more directly involved in ensuring that prisoners were not exposed to unconstitutional conditions. The ACLU's successes continued throughout the 1980s and early into the next decade.

Indeed, by the beginning of the 1990s, nearly all states faced litigation for inadequate prison health care, and many of these cases have resulted in court orders or consent decrees requiring substantial remedies on the part of prison administrators. Susan Sturm reported:

> As of January 1993, forty states plus the District of Columbia, Puerto Rico, and the Virgin Islands were under court order to reduce overcrowding and/or eliminate unconstitutional conditions of confinement. Twenty-five percent of all jails in the United States were under court order to reduce crowding in 1990, and thirty percent were under court order to improve conditions of confinement. In 1989, seven percent of the nation's 422 facilities detaining ten percent of all incarcerated youngsters were operating under consent decrees.[10]

In the decade after Judge Johnson first declared Alabama's prisons "unfit for human habitation,"[11] prison conditions in the state had made some important, though still very modest, improvements. After a tour in 1986, Larry Yackle cautiously recounted:

> The physical facilities were improved, but primarily at the level of housekeeping. Even the new prisons in the north showed signs of wear; in the

south, the threat of slipping back to ruin was palpable . . . The space requirements fixed by Judge Johnson had never been met.[12]

Despite Yackle's misgivings, it is undeniable that the conclusion of Malcolm Feeley and Edward Rubin in their important study of the history
of prison reform in the United States is truer of the situation today than
of the situation only decades ago, when U.S. jails and prisons operated in
all but the absence of judicial oversight: "Conditions and practices are
much improved and the constitutionalization of the process assures
that these improvements are likely to be permanent."[13] Yet, echoing
Yackle's concerns, Feeley and Rubin remain cautiously optimistic:

> The mission of prisons and jails remains safety and security by means of
> a tight system of control. Judicial reform has, on balance, enhanced the
> ability of officials to pursue this mission: They are now more, not less, ef-
> fective and efficient.[14]

In addition to the successes in the courts, it is important to take a
critical look at the important gains prisoner rights activists have
achieved, especially in regards to the treatment of HIV+ prisoners in
the post-PLRA era.

Social Activism and HIV+ Prisoner Rights

In his important book *Ideology and the New Social Movements,* sociologist Alan Scott advances a conception of social movements as potentially powerful political organizations that can pressure other institutions to integrate their main interests.[15] Scott's conception, as
sociologist and leading prisoner rights activist Rachel Maddow has recently demonstrated, is especially prescient for understanding the
work of contemporary activists. Given the "toughening" of the federal judiciary and the dramatic undercutting of prisoner rights as embodied by the PLRA, activists have played an especially critical role in
persuading prison officials to recognize the importance of addressing
the HIV/AIDS crisis behind bars. Maddow's extensive interviews
with activists and other key actors involved in the movement demonstrate their remarkable achievements. Maddow writes:

[P]rison officials have not precluded HIV/AIDS activists' access to prisons and prisoners. Prisoners living with (or at risk for) HIV/AIDS have been both the subjects of outsiders' advocacy, and the agents of advocacy themselves. There has not been an overwhelming backlash against HIV/AIDS activism in prisons, and prison administrators have engaged co-operatively with HIV/AIDS activists to a greater extent than they have with other prisoners' advocates.[16]

According to Maddow, HIV/AIDS activists have most dramatically integrated their interests into the prison setting by convincing some prison bureaucrats that activists and prisoners alike are "experts" who can play important roles in the education and treatment of HIV+ prisoners.[17]

Activists have doubtlessly played a critical role in building support networks for HIV+ prisoners and, in turn, have empowered prisoners to play active roles in the education of their fellow prisoners. But within the broader activist movement concerning HIV/AIDS, prisoner issues have long been marginalized. Sociologist Brett Stockdill's trenchant analysis of the movement in his book *Activism against AIDS* demonstrates—through numerous interviews with activists from Chicago, New York, and Los Angeles—the long-standing challenges faced by the national movement called the AIDS Coalition to Unleash Power (ACT UP), as it seeks to have prison issues taken seriously. At the core of the disconnect is the inability of the majority of ACT UP members to see beyond the "us and them" ideology that drives present-day "tough on crime" initiatives. Stockdill observes:

I discovered that AIDS activists are not immune to stereotypical images of prisoners. Mainstream AIDS activists were frequently caught up in the "law and order," "three strikes and you're out" mentality that has guided our society's approach to crime and punishment in recent decades.[18]

This intramovement struggle, which sociologist Aldon Morris calls "partial oppositional consciousness,"[19] has obviously made things more difficult for HIV+ prisoner activists. For one, they have not received from the movement the kind of financial support needed to implement their ambitious treatment and education agendas behind bars. Nevertheless, this relatively small collective of passionate activists have played a vitally important role in the recent struggle.

Honing Movement Tactics

Although prisoner rights activists were not immediately focused on HIV/AIDS behind bars, their efforts at building national networks around prisoner health issues would prove invaluable for strategizing in later years. Beginning in the mid-1980s, Ellen Barry and her organization Legal Services for Prisoners with Children created both the National Network for Women in Prison (NNWP) and the National Roundtable on Women in Prison, an annual conference that brought together fifty-five activists from across the United States to talk and strategize about issues affecting incarcerated mothers and their children. In 1989, nearly two hundred people from around the United States, Canada, and Mexico, attended the conference, and the conference theme expanded from incarcerated mothers to all women in prison. By 1993, the National Roundtable on Women in Prison, in its seventh year, was held at American University's Washington College of Law in Washington, D.C. By this time, the NNWP had become something far more than just an organization that sponsored an annual conference. Barry explains:

> The Roundtable was a forum for community activists and advocates and members of the network . . . Regional representatives met at this conference and began to function as a Board . . . Angela Davis was a keynote speaker . . . The NNWP reached a new level of sophistication and visibility with the development of a professional logo and a presence in the U.S. capital.[20]

Perhaps most important for HIV+ prisoners, the conferencing, public education campaigns, and other organizational tactics honed by the NNWP have been integrated with litigation strategies. Indeed, Stockdill's analysis of members of the ACT UP/Prison Issue Committee in Chicago demonstrates that activism alone, without the threat of legal subpoena, proved an uphill battle. Although activists at California's state prison at Vacaville had more success on this front,[21] the most important breakthroughs ultimately took place when activists and lawyers began working together cooperatively.

In 1994, having witnessed the creation of a sophisticated network of prison lawyers, activists, and prisoners, Ellen Barry and colleagues waged the campaign on behalf of HIV+ women prisoners in California. Barry described to me the decision to move forward with what would become a sweeping class action lawsuit, *Shumate v. Wilson*.

> We were shocked about how bad the care was. They used Tylenol 3 for the pain of breast cancer or AIDS. People just cannot deal with that level of pain and inhumanity. So Charisse Shumate became the lead plaintive. She was extremely close with the group of women who were HIV-positive who were leading the effort. Fortunately, we were able to slip it in under the wire, before the PLRA passed.[22]

The *Shumate* litigation proved to be an important means for organizing prisoner rights lawyers and activists on the outside.

Barry and her colleagues organized a support coalition that brought together lawyers, HIV/AIDS street activists, and members of the few northern California prison organizations (e.g., California Prison Focus and the Pelican Bay Information Project) for a series of meetings held in the offices of a downtown San Francisco law firm.[23] Participants discussed the *Shumate* suit and planned demonstrations and media strategies to create a climate of support. They also discussed broader issues of prison conditions, prison litigation, and the overall movement for California prison reform. The lawsuit and the resources of the lawyers involved provided an important catalyst for a movement-building and movement-sustaining event—as well as providing important material capital, such as meeting space, a minute taker, photocopying equipment, food, and other amenities—when resource-strapped nonlawyer activists alone may not have been able to do so. The meetings also spawned the formation of new groups, including the California Coalition for Women Prisoners, an active nonlegal advocacy group made up mostly of activist women in the San Francisco Bay Area and formed by members of the *Shumate* coalition and others in the month following the initial meeting at the downtown law office.[24]

Losing Ground

In light of continued overcrowding, the stubborn secrecy of jail and prison bureaucracies, the difficult roadblocks of the PLRA, and the pervasive amorality associated with captive institutions (explored in more detail in chapter 6), the challenges confronting activist groups focused on monitoring conditions of confining HIV+ prisoners has become a Sisyphean task. As will become clearer in the responses of numerous prisoner rights lawyers and activists I have interviewed, activism in this era of increasingly catastrophic penal institutions is often characterized by desperation, frustration, and loss. Even in California, the organizing efforts around the *Shumate* litigation would prove invaluable as a last hope for those women prisoners needlessly suffering and dying behind bars, but overcrowding, the severe deterioration of prison conditions, and indifference among prison personnel made things increasingly difficult to affect change in the state's penal institutions.

Sociologist Nancy Stoller's analysis of access to health care by California's HIV+ women prisoners sheds important light on a pervasive indifference on the part of prison staff to prisoner suffering and death in California's women's prisons.[25] In an analysis of 1,269 files of women's complaints from three prisons between 1996 and 1999—including files used in the *Shumate* litigation—Stoller found that a common complaint among women prisoners with HIV/AIDS concerned lack of access to proper medications. As will be come clearer in chapter 6, assessment by Stoller and colleagues hinted at a catastrophic breakdown in each of the institution's medical care systems. Like the male HIV+ population at Limestone, California's women prisoners with HIV/AIDS were routinely denied close and consistent care. The stories from Stoller's report provide chilling evidence of serious lapses in care.

> Ellen Blair has waited two weeks for HIV meds. She has had very little appetite and difficulty eating. She reports that staff forbids prisoners from taking showers and refuses to assist in sponge baths. Often they lock her in or out of her room, limiting her mobility . . . Christina Sosa suffered immensely. She was confined to her bed and completely immobile except for slight control over her left arm. She suffered from wasting

disease and neuropathy . . . Her [emergency] call button did not always work. When it did staff routinely took a long time to respond.[26]

Although Stoller's report does not attend to the dynamics that help to explain these institutional failures, her analysis strongly suggests an amoral culture that enabled prison medical staff to normalize prisoner suffering and deaths. In chapter 6, I will explore a more detailed "anatomy of institutional failure" that emerged at Limestone prison over a five-year period, between 1999 and 2003. But it is first necessary to explore the challenges faced by those in the trenches of America's catastrophic jails and prisons today.

Voices from the Inside

The contemporary struggle for the humane treatment of HIV+ prisoners has, to dramatically understate the problem, been an uphill battle. Lawyers and activists on the ground today are faced with increasingly desperate situations, often involving the life and death of those they work with. As will become clear in the remainder of this chapter, prison overcrowding and deteriorating prison conditions serve as an important backdrop for the stories the lawyers and activists tell. While I pay special attention to the impact of the PLRA on contemporary prisoner rights lawyering and activism, several of the stories presented will testify to systems of medical care that are profoundly inadequate. I begin with an in-depth look at the lived experiences of prisoner rights lawyers and advocates in the post-PLRA era.

In the Shadow of the PLRA

The PLRA has had negative effects on prisoner rights advocacy concerning chronically ill prisoners, has created new and more daunting challenges for institutional change, and has made prisoner rights lawyers and activists less hopeful that litigation can result in meaningful change.[27] To explore these observations in more detail, this chapter turns to the specific experiential accounts of prisoner lawyers and activists—that is, those fighting for lives on the inside. The accounts of advocates from around the United States reveal that the PLRA has created dramatic institutional roadblocks to holding penal institutions accountable. Coupled with the acceptance of waste management as the primary goal of state officials in charge of managing dramatically overcrowded penal institutions in the United States today, the PLRA has made the vitally important watchdog function of prisoner law organizations far more challenging.

At the broadest level, the capping of attorneys' fees mandated by the PLRA seems to have made it increasingly difficult for prison law offices to stay economically afloat. Of the organizations that do continue to operate, attorneys are forced to work longer hours for less pay. Turning to the stories of advocates, it is clear that the bureaucratic red tape of the PLRA has made it more difficult to address serious problems with prisoners' health care until it is often too late. Obvious lapses in care that could have been immediately addressed are left routinely to escalate into life-threatening crises.

Depending on their institutional roles, the accounts of activists touch on, to varying degrees, the challenges of the post-PLRA world of advocacy. For example, directors of organizations tend to focus on broader managerial problems, such as decreases in funding. The presentation of the respondents in this chapter focuses on an important conception for other studies of law and social change—namely, the institutional context.

The Institutional Effects of Antirights Law

As has been discussed by Lauren Edelman, the passage of a law like the PLRA requires one to pay particular attention to the "complexity of the organizational reaction to environmental changes," since "formal structures that become institutionalized may be relatively unaffected by—or at least slow to respond to—a subsequent loss of public or legal support."[28] The PLRA is an interesting case in this respect. Obviously, penal institutions are uniquely authoritarian captive organizations, which legal scholar and sociologist James Jacobs long ago observed are particularly stubborn to court mandates. But the PLRA is a uniquely antirights law. Indeed, the following accounts illustrate how a formal law can actually embolden institutions against those who attempt to challenge or reform them.

Advocates in Leadership Roles

LEN ERICKSON

Len Erickson,[29] a former director of a prisoner legal project on the East Coast, describes how the PLRA has led to the shutdown of many prisoner rights projects across the United States.

> The PLRA has influenced everything, or at least, it does among those who are still able to stay in business after the PLRA. And there aren't many of them. The PLRA narrowed the causes of action even further and limited the fees that you could recover even if you won. So, now you have fewer meritorious suits, legally meritorious suits, and less money even if you win. All around the country, little prisoner law shops are going out of business. My prisoner shop is still up and running, but that is, if I may say so, thanks to creative leadership. I mean, if you do the equivalent of a Nexis search and look at how many of them there were ten years ago, you know the local prisoner rights projects, they're all gone now.[30]

It is difficult to challenge Len Erickson's grim assessment in an era that has become increasingly and aggressively against prisoner rights. One clear indicator of this bent is the massive federal and state spending on prison construction and simultaneous defunding of prisoner services.[31] As the next account makes clear, even longtime national organizations committed to prisoner rights have experienced dramatic cuts in resources.

ALEXANDRA MICHAELS

An advocate for a national prison legal services organization, Alexandra Michaels describes the impact of the PLRA on her organization.

> When it became apparent that PLRA was going to be passed, the first impact that it had on my office was that the organization decided to cut the budget by about a quarter . . . The projects are self supporting—and we were primarily supporting ourselves with attorneys fees—and it would be so difficult to win new cases because the fee provisions of PLRA drastically cut the availability of attorney's fees; the organization correctly an-

ticipated that we would have substantially less income. So, the first impact was that there were cuts in staff and cuts in programs.

The impact of the PLRA has also negatively impacted Michaels's work routine. Specifically, she contrasts her work schedule as a new public interest lawyer with her present schedule post-PLRA.

The second impact was when it really became just the standard thing to work sixty- to seventy-hour weeks on a routine basis. I mean, that's what you did during trial. When I went into public interest law it was supposed to be good, as unlike working for a firm, you got regular time off. Now, my standard week I'm working seven days a week. And that just sort of happens with PLRA. It also happened in the point of my life where my kids were growing up and I could do it in a way that I couldn't have done it earlier.

Regardless of how many hours she works, fighting the PLRA proves extremely difficult for Michaels, if not impossible.

In any event, we lost a lot of cases, and we spent huge amounts of time organizing the plan of bargain, getting the standard briefs done, and fighting PLRA to the extent that we could . . . It really has made the litigation much more difficult to do. It now literally means that cases that were won once don't necessarily stay won.

BARRY ECKHART

Barry Eckhart, a prisoner rights lawyer from the eastern United States, expounds on the tension (alluded to by Alexandra Michaels) between the personal and the professional. Specifically, Eckhart describes how both the substandard conditions within the prison and the broader cutbacks in funding for prisoner legal services have negatively impacted not only lawyers' ability to help individual prisoners but their ability to file class action lawsuits.

The mayor really cut back our funding. We felt like we were fortunate when we got funding for a couple of years, but then the sources dried up. So we lost a paralegal and that is a huge impact. We have dealt with literally thousands of inmates and we have been literally overwhelmed by the real tension between helping individuals and moving a class action, and we are really stumbling on that. People call up and want to have direct and immediate needs and that's a real tension when it is totally removed from the class-action. We don't have adequate resources to really do both effectively, and so I think that has caused a tremendous amount of delay in our litigation.

Eckhart describes how the inhumanity of prison life only complicates efforts at meaningful advocacy on behalf of sick prisoners.

People who are incarcerated have a myriad of problems. We are often the only ones they have to deal with some of those problems, and some of them we can do something about and some of them we can't. How many times have I spent on the phone—but I think it is important, because prisoners have almost no power.

In Eckhart's experience, many prisoners feel so oppressed by the prison system that they actually sabotage their own health as a form of protest.

The only power they often have is the refusal power. They are angry because they wouldn't let them see a specialist, so what do they do: "I am going to refuse all of my medication," or "I am going to refuse to see the doctor because he is insulting to me." So this refusal of care is sometimes the only power that they have. Constantly, I am confronted with that. Then I do counseling of how this may be counterproductive. I understand their rage; it is even justified, but is refusal really effective for their own health care? So, we are also social workers and counselors. I am dealing with their medical care, but this officer is harassing them, or they are not safe, and so you deal with all those problems. Do you deal with them as a human being? Do you deal with them because often this population has a lot of social needs that they need your representation on? All of those things can be terribly time-consuming. So it is a constant compromise between providing any of those services or all of those services and doing your big class-action litigation.

ELIZABETH SAWYER

A longtime prisoner rights lawyer and activist from the West Coast, Elizabeth Sawyer echoes Barry Lawrence's sentiments but also argues that personal injury damages in prisoner rights cases are typically exceedingly difficult to litigate. Specifically, when telling the story of a mistreated prisoner infected with AIDS, Sawyer describes how she and her fellow litigators decided not to pursue personal injury damages.

> We chose not to go for the damages in her case, and I think we should have, but we chose other cases to move forward. In part we chose to do this because of the way that personal injury law played out, and the difficulty of selling these cases to personal injury lawyers who do not want to deal with prisoners—things like having advanced AIDS and being left in excruciating pain with shingles or something like that. But can be it proved that that is a personal injury case? Well, no, what we really need to do is get immediate relief for the women. So we may have to choose between the common strategies, or maybe what is really important to her at that point is not so much getting money damages but getting her to the hospital. So it is very, very difficult and painful.

Sawyer explains that even when her organization wins a class action lawsuit, the challenge continues.

> There is a tendency to think that if you win a lawsuit it will all go away. But it doesn't. You get corrections to agree to change one thing, and then the very next day they are out to erode that as much as they can.

Sawyer's decades of experience working with women prisoners lead her to conclude:

> You will hear it differently from other people who feel they are more balanced about it, but I take it from what I see, and I have interviewed literally thousands of women. I feel like the truth kind of emerges, maybe not from one or two interviews, but if you interview enough people, and they are all saying the same thing—or variations of the same thing—you probably have something there.

Attorneys and Activists

SALLY REDMOND

The preceding accounts of individuals in leadership roles in prisoner rights organizations from around the United States highlight the difficulties of litigation post-PLRA. At the same time, these leaders talk about an increasingly pessimistic future for prisoner advocacy. The following account, from activist Sally Redmond, sheds light on how the burdens of the PLRA have made attorneys less available to engage in grassroots activism, especially the coordination of all-important public awareness campaigns.

Redmond, a longtime prisoner rights activist from a West Coast organization, believes that the PLRA—by making it more difficult for lawyers to share important information with activists—has a directly negative effect on prisoner rights activism. Specifically, she argues that by creating extra layers of bureaucratic red tape and diverting resources, the PLRA has cut dramatically into the time lawyers have available to bring important media attention to activist organizations.

> I always thought that having both lawyers and activists working together is more effective than just focusing on litigation alone. But part of it really is the PLRA. The lawyers try to do what they could within the confines of the federal legislation and stuff but, because they are so tied up in red tape, they are less able to give you a hook to interest the media—stuff to have demonstrations around.

The institutional inertia created by the PLRA's red tape has doubtlessly made the task of prisoner rights activists and attorneys more daunting. There is simply less time for lawyers and activists to work together.

CHRISTINA DYER

Beyond the aforementioned negative changes to prisoner rights advocacy, Christina Dyer, a lawyer and activist from a prisoner rights organization on the West Coast, suggests that the PLRA has led prison officials to become far more lax about meeting court-imposed mandates involving adequate health care. While we cannot know how widespread this chilling effect has been, it is clear that in many of the nation's penal institutions, the deregulating of prisoner rights protections has resulted in serious problems concerning the treatment of the dangerously ill. In a chilling contrast to three decades of prison reform culminating in the Civil Rights of Institutionalized Persons Act (CRIPA) of 1983,[32] the PLRA (set against a backdrop of extreme prisoner overcrowding and the attendant focus on waste management) reveals a veritable culture of indifference on the part of medical staff to seriously ill prisoners.

While this observation needs to be assessed in the context of particular institutional dynamics, it is clear that in the early 1980s, there was more attention paid to the grievous conditions in the nation's jails and prisons than there is now. Specifically, there were clear objectives to the passage of CRIPA: dozens of cases of prisoner abuse and neglect mobilized Congress to become more actively involved in the operations of the nation's penal institutions. But such a mandate becomes highly problematic when it is largely undercut by the PLRA and mass incarceration policies. By contrast to the PLRA, CRIPA only required a prisoner to exhaust all administrative remedies if the prison was certified as having grievance procedures that were "plain, speedy, and effective."[33]

Dyer tells a chilling story of the powerlessness of post-PLRA prisoner rights lawyers to challenge substandard medical care. Dyer begins with a story of the circumstances leading up to the death of an important activist prisoner, herself infected with both HIV and hepatitis C. Apparently this prisoner received retaliation by prison health officials for contesting her grossly substandard care.

> There was an activist prisoner who I worked with for four years who is actually in pretty good health, and she had HIV, but she was non-symptomatic. And her viral-load was virtually nonexistent even though she was on medication, and she is basically just fine with her HIV health, but she was also infected with hepatitis C. She had very pronounced signs of liver disease and was getting sicker and sicker. She argued—and we couldn't prove this element of it—she thought that in response to how she was advocating for other prisoners for their health care, the chief medical officer at the prison she was at wanted to *get rid of her and get her out of the institution.* So he had her pulled out of her room and sent her across the street to a different prison, allegedly for having tuberculosis. She was put into isolation and given tuberculosis medications which are highly liver-toxic. Anyway, she didn't have any signs or symptoms of having TB. She thought, and I would agree, that he probably did this to get her out of the way, but she went into liver failure as a result of these medications and died. Before she died she was sent back to the other prison, and that chief

medical officer then tried to cover up her condition and was trying to say that she wasn't sick when in fact she was sick.

In a disturbing aside to her story, Dyer reveals how the PLRA suddenly became "inapplicable" in this case.

The day after she died, we got a letter postmarked and dated after she was already dead telling us that her condition was under control and she was fine; the letter was from that chief medical officer. He also then—we suspected that she was dying and we were trying to get her family to have a special permission for bereavement visits to see her quickly and they denied that. So she died without her family being able to say goodbye, and [the prison] also tried to cover up the death. But we "got around" the Prison Litigation Reform Act because she was dead. So obviously, under the new system, she was an "okay plaintiff" because she was dead. We sued on her family's behalf for negligence and intentional infliction of emotional distress on them and [for] the doctor's failure to admit that she was near death. But her family was not prisoners, so we could actually file a lawsuit.

This experience reminds Dyer that for prisoner rights lawyers, such as herself, this case is not an anomalous occurrence—perhaps less so since the passage of the PLRA.

We just see so many of these things on a regular basis that should be lawsuits, where the time limits aren't met, or we just know the exhaustion is never going to be met, or there is no way that we can find an attorney who will take a financial risk to take the cases. It is really heartbreaking and it is something that we constantly see now.

If the PLRA has hindered effective advocacy, it is not surprising that sick prisoners are paying the price—sometimes, as Dyer's story makes clear, with their lives. The remaining accounts presented in this chapter shed light on the institutional conditions that lead to increased suffering and preventable deaths among HIV-infected prisoners post-PLRA. The final four accounts thus serve as a very preliminary primer to the more in-depth analysis of preventable deaths at Limestone prison presented in chapter 6.

Susan Billy is an ex-prisoner, activist, and paralegal with a nonprofit prison law project on the East Coast. A story she tells of a fellow prisoner elucidates the inability of prison health care systems to address the specialized needs of HIV-infected prisoners.

> Let's see, there was one female who was HIV positive. And she, um, had to do what they call "wasting." Wasting is when you lose more than ten pounds in a year. And she had lost, oh God, I would guess thirty or forty pounds. And it was because of the fact that the doctors in the prison setting give everybody the same medicine regimen. Nobody has a specified regimen for themselves. They just give everybody the same things and hope that it works. So people were getting sick, and not responding well to the medications that they were receiving because they were all getting the same thing.

Billy also describes a second prisoner's death as treated in a cold, bureaucratic fashion by prison doctors.

> There was a female who died who was very, very sick. And she went to the infirmary and they told her she was fine. So, she went back to her unit. Well, the inmates ended up carrying her back to the infirmary. And the doctors acted as if nothing was wrong. They locked her in a room in the back and she died. They just let her die in there.

MANUEL COLON

An ex-prisoner and activist from the Northeast, Manuel Colon describes the emotionally and physically cruel and unusual conditions experienced by HIV-infected prisoners post-PLRA. In answering the question "What are some recent challenges you have faced as a prisoner rights activist," he described a recent visit to a state prison's new special housing units (SHUs),[34] which he calls "high-tech dungeons."

> There are about eight of these self-contained prisons that they built on the grounds of already existing prisons. And they cost twelve million dollars to build. I refer to them as a "high-tech dungeon." There are two people locked in a cell for twenty-three hours. They are so contained that

they have a shower in the cell, they have a door that opens in the back of the cell that leads into this little area that they call a "dog kennel."

Colon further describes how even HIV-infected prisoners may be confined in SHUs.

> Oh yeah, HIV+ prisoners are there. I think it is so damaging psychologically. You know, the mental, emotional, and spiritual damage of the people confined under these conditions. It's horrible.

Colon's account suggests that a heightened focus on isolation trumps care. Rather than an emphasis on specialized therapeutic care, the overcrowded institution Colon works in as a prisoner rights advocate utilizes SHU's. Like Limestone's "Thunderdorm," these "dog kennels" are places of containment and control. They are zones of disciplinc that cast a far-reaching shadow over the institution. In them, chronically ill and, as a recent report from Human Rights Watch makes abundantly clear, mentally debilitated prisoners are rendered depersonalized—indeed, dehumanized—units.[35]

HEATHER MICHELLE SAMUELS

Heather Michelle Samuels, an AIDS activist and prison hospice volunteer from a southern state, describes her first experience as a social worker assigned to a hospital that serves the medical needs of state prisoners. Like the stories of Billy and Colon, Samuels's account is one of a prison system that is largely indifferent to sick prisoners.

> My first contact was working as a hospital medical social worker at our city hospital. And all inmates are brought here for their health care. They are shackled to their beds no matter how sick they are. So, my consciousness really got raised there, and got me involved in working on behalf of the inmates. I was working with people who couldn't even move because of the shackles, which is a distinct danger if there was a fire, or if they shared a room with an aggressive or psychotic patient.

Samuels tells a story of "one of the two worst things" she saw at the hospital.

And one of the two worst things I saw was when a shackled inmate who they needed to resuscitate, and they had to wait for the guard to come and unshackle him because it was metal—well, he died. And that was such an absolutely horrifying thing to think that maybe it would've been different. And then I had another patient who had very advanced AIDS and was slowly losing his mental faculties as well as his ability to walk or move his arms in any way. And they insisted that he had to be shackled to the bed; he was totally confused. He did not get better, and the hospital wanted to send him back to the jail, and we tried, my supervisor and I tried to get him released so we could place him, because we thought he was probably terminal but the jail would not release him. So, he was instead sent back to jail, and we thought that the jail would say, "We can't manage somebody this sick" and release him, which they often do and send him to the hospital, or, if they send him to the hospital, they would then release him from there. But he was basically dumped there in the jail. And they kept him for about three weeks; when he came back to the hospital he also died. He died in custody still shackled to the bed.

It is tempting to interpret Samuels's story as one involving a "few bad apples" responsible for the cruel treatment that led to the death of these prisoners. But it is far more likely that the men who chained the dying prisoners to their beds were "simply following orders." To understand how typically "good" people—in this case, prison guards—carry out such dirty, amoral work, one must attend to the penal institution's overriding security mandate. Such situations must, moreover, not be seen as separate from the present sociohistorical moment, which is characterized by an aggressive security-centered approach.

WALTER SPENCE

Each of the preceding stories reveal how a growing lack of institutional accountability has led to dysfunctional penal bureaucracies that break down at the expense of HIV-infected prisoners, with obvious consequences for their health and sometimes their lives. This situation is only made worse when considering HIV-infected prisoners who are unable to read or write. The stories of prisoner lawyers and activists describe such prisoners as not only subjected to grossly substandard prison health care but, because of illiteracy, at even greater disadvantage when it comes to understanding their disease and what treatments to demand from health care staff.

An ex-prisoner and longtime activist from the Northwest, Walter Spence describes an experience with an HIV-infected prisoner who was unable to read or write and was also blind.

> Well, he had only been diagnosed for two weeks, but he obviously had HIV for a long time. He gets diagnosed, put in the hospital, the orderlies are inmates, they won't even touch him and he's got no pillow, he's lying on this little thing and can't get comfortable. He's like, "I just can't get comfortable." And I'm like, "What are they doing to you?" And he goes, "I know nothing about it." He couldn't read or write, and he didn't have any way to get any information except from what they told him about his disease. They gave him no medications or anything. And the thing is he can't see, so they send him to the optometrist, and the optometrist says, "We haven't seen this in a prisoner with AIDS in ten years." I mean, there are drugs to take care of this kind of stuff. But of course he's not getting them. He's not getting any care, and he loses his eyesight over it and it's awful. And on top of all that, he's gonna die soon.

Perhaps more than any other story presented in here, Spence's account elucidates how an ill-equipped, disorganized prison medical system leads to catastrophic institutional failure. The case of an older prisoner with advanced disease exposes the institution's grossly inadequate system of preventative care. Rather than monitor this man's condition, his health care providers left him untreated until a catastrophe ensued. What was likely a situation that could have been prevented with a reliable medical assessment and consistent monitoring was left to fester. The man lost his vision as a result of a lack of care and was sent to an obviously dismayed vision specialist, whose diagnosis of not having seen someone in such condition in ten years is about more than the prisoner losing his vision. As Spence observes, this neglected prisoner with AIDS was categorized by staff as someone that was "gonna die soon."

Confronting Prisoners' Health Post-PLRA

Translating the mandates of prisoner rights activism and litigation into genuine institutional reform has always been an uphill battle for judges, lawyers, and activists. Even in the days of a more activist judiciary—indeed, at the height of the civil rights movement in America—the law has only been able to make moderately positive changes in the treatment of prisoners, including those with chronic illnesses. In this age of exploding penal populations and dwindling state budgets, the situation has only worsened.

In the next two chapters, I turn to an intensive case study of HIV-related deaths at Limestone prison between 1999 and 2003. Chapter 5 explores the litigation strategy employed by the Southern Center for Human Rights (SCHR) on behalf of Limestone's HIV+ prisoner class. Specifically, I investigate how SCHR learned of the case, what uniquely daunting challenges the PLRA created, and how SCHR confronted catastrophic institutional failure at Limestone. The discussion of how the imperatives of punishment and cost cutting on the part of political and penal elites conflicts with the reform-minded goals of prisoner rights advocates provides critical context for the analysis of *Leatherwood v. Campbell*. In chapter 6, I turn to an investigation of how mass incarceration and the consequences of cost cutting led to a profound breakdown in the care of Limestone's most gravely ill prisoners. Specifically, I explore how such breakdown led to what I call a "zone of lethal abandonment."

CHAPTER 5   The Challenges

of *Leatherwood*

It was the summer of 2002. Josh Lipman had just finished law school
and was to begin his first job as an attorney with the Southern Center
for Human Rights (SCHR). What he did not know was that he would
be in charge of his first case, Limestone, before he even arrived at
SCHR's downtown Atlanta offices. He explains, "I remember that I
was driving on my way to the airport and [that] there was going to be
a conference call in the afternoon about the conditions for HIV+
prisoners in Alabama and that there was a horrible situation occurring there."[1] Since accumulating experiences as an SCHR intern assisting Tamara Serwer with the Fulton County Jail case in 2000 (see
chapter 2) and, ultimately, finding some satisfaction in the settlement
reached in that case, Lipman did not hesitate in responding. "I said
'Okay, I'll be there,'" he remembers, "and I got on a plane and got
there twenty minutes before the meeting." At the meeting, he learned
that Limestone was a far more complex beast than the Fulton County
Jail case. Whereas Serwer had the time to persuade Fulton County
officials that it was in their interest to address the institution's failure
to provide HIV+ prisoners protease inhibitors, Limestone presented
SCHR with a host of pressing issues.

Lipman learned that approximately two hundred HIV+ prisoners at Limestone were currently living in a decrepit warehouse used previously, in the late 1990s, to house Alabama's chain gang. Dorm 16 (the official name of the facility) was, however, not the HIV+ prisoners first home at Limestone. While there is speculation that the prisoners were moved as retaliation for a previously failed class action, one thing was certain: Dorm 16 and the Health Care Unit (HCU) were far from adequate. Lipman describes his first visit in the fall of 2002 as follows:

> The warehouse is literally falling apart around them. The roof has been collapsing, and the rain was leaking in. There are rats and spiders that bite the inmates. They do all of their cooking and living in this warehouse because they are not allowed to associate with the rest of the prison population. The warehouse is located on the other side of the prison from the HCU, so during emergencies, it can take thirty to forty minutes for inmates to be brought there from Dorm 16. I mean, I learned that numerous inmates had actually died on the route.

Lipman's initial observation points to a particularly important feature of institutional failure at Limestone. Specifically, the distance from Dorm 16 to the HCU reveals an important spatial dimension of prisoner suffering and preventable deaths. I explore this and other related issues in more detail in chapter 6.

Assisting Josh Lipman was Lisa Zahren, an SCHR investigator who had also worked on the Fulton County Jail case. Zahren had been to Limestone previously, so she knew full well what this case entailed. She first learned about the prison after receiving two letters from prisoners incarcerated at Alabama's infamously overcrowded and oppressive Madison County Jail. One of the men who contacted Zahren was arrested on a probation violation and held first at Madison County Jail. Upon discovery of his HIV status, he was shipped immediately to Dorm 16; Alabama law requires that all HIV+ male prisoners be housed at Limestone prison. In a shocking discovery, Zahren's investigation uncovered that the man's probation violation was, in fact, dropped. In short, the prison bureaucracy allowed for the incarceration of an innocent man because of his disability. Zahren recounts:

When he went to the county jail, he told them, "I have all of these expensive HIV medications, and I need to see my HIV doctor." And within a week they violated his probation and shipped him off to Limestone. Without any due process! I mean, you give up a lot of your rights when you're on probation. So he gets sent to Limestone; he sits there for a couple of months in limbo. But he keeps writing to Madison County Jail saying, "I have this new charge, and I need to find out what the status of it is, whether or not I've actually been indicted, and if I have an attorney." And he finally gets a letter back saying the new charge was dropped! So the probation violation that he got sent to Limestone for was completely dropped. But because of the Department of Corrections total lack of management, he got stuck in limbo there and actually ended up serving time.

Zahren's phrase "lack of management" is important to understanding the plight of this man. It is very likely that no one individual employee of the Alabama Department of Corrections (ADOC) intended for the man to be wrongfully incarcerated. Instead, the system's absence of services meant that an HIV+ individual who lacked an attorney was forced to serve time in the deplorable conditions of Dorm 16. In Alabama, once an indigent suspect is found to be HIV+, the official policy is one of targeted transfer. The policy had been in place for many years and thus was likely never questioned by ADOC staff. Fortunately, this man was able to write an all-important letter to SCHR. Indeed, from the prisoner's perspective, the ability to send a letter to the outside world had taken on an awesome meaning. For many prisoners, it is a last-ditch effort to get the treatment they often desperately need; sometimes, their lives depend on it.

Similar to how she learned about the Madison County Jail debacle, Zahren's first insight into just how dire the circumstances had become inside Dorm 16 came from prisoner's letters, beginning in early 2000. Perhaps most shocking, she learned about a plague of boils that was infecting Limestone's HIV+ population. Many of the men were covered with boils anywhere from the size of a golf ball to a grapefruit. The boils would grow to a head, burst, and then drain for days all over their clothing and bedding. SCHR knew that this situation itself was so serious that it needed to be addressed immediately, so they contacted Limestone's medical provider.

Naphcare, a Birmingham-based health care provider, had taken over all of Limestone's medical care in 2000. Like ADOC, Naphcare did not return any of SCHR's phone calls. Finally, in a brazen act of mitigating destructiveness, there was a response: ADOC claimed that the boils were only mosquito bites and that the health care providers were on top of the situation. But Zahren had seen with her own eyes that these were not mosquito bites.

> I mean, I'm talking to one of the prisoners there, and he has this golf-ball-sized boil on his arm, and I said, "What is that thing?" He was like, "Oh, everyone has these." And it was this horrible infection that just tore through the place: out of the two hundred guys, probably eighty have these things. And they're terribly painful, you get a fever, and they just ooze with pus. So this prisoner is telling me all these stories about people having other people pop them for them. At that time—I don't know if you still can—but you could actually order a sewing needle from Limestone's store. What I learned was that these needles were being purchased and used to pop these; the men were sharing the needles to pop these wounds.

All the signs of a dire medical emergency were present. How could the prison's medical staff have allowed the boil outbreak to have occurred in the first place? Wouldn't the disturbingly widespread use of sewing needles among the population send out a red flag that something more serious was happening? SCHR would not wait to find the answers to these questions. At the time that this disturbing news first became known, the organization aggressively sought more information. Lipman contacted some of the top HIV experts from all across the United States. Based on their discussions, Lipman and colleagues concluded that the plague of boils was the result of a widespread staph infection. But this insight was just the tip of a very large and disturbing iceberg. Lipman learned that for many years, anywhere between fourteen and sixteen of Limestone's HIV+ prisoners were dying each year.

ADOC Hires Naphcare

It is clear from an investigative report conducted by *Birmingham News* journalist Carla Crowder that cost cutting was ADOC's main objective in hiring Naphcare.[2] In 2000, the Alabama governor, Democrat Donald Siegelman, a vocal advocate for harsh sentencing policies, championed the idea that prisoners should be required to pay for their incarceration; he advocated the revitalization of Alabama's infamous chain gangs. It is not surprising that he, like many "tough on crime" governors across the United States, turned his sights to dramatically cutting health care costs behind bars.

Despite an Alabama prison health official's demand, reported by Crowder, that any contract should stipulate that the provider "match industry standards laid out by the National Commission on Correctional Health Care (NCCHC), which accredits prison and jail health systems,"[3] Governor Siegelman devised a way to hire not only the cheapest but by far the least qualified bidder for the contract: Birmingham-based Naphcare. While none of the four companies that bid on the contract met NCCHC criteria, Naphcare did not even meet qualifications to submit a bid. Most glaringly, Naphcare lacked experience. the company had never worked with a prison population of at least twenty thousand, and it had absolutely no experience with mental health care.

A leading Alabama prison health official told Crowder that when he raised concerns, he "was told point blank by [the governor's attorney] to shut up."[4] Crowder reports that when this same official talked with the corrections commissioner at the time, he was told, "We are not going to do anything to make the Governor look bad."[5] Instead of setting out specific industry care standards, the contract focused almost entirely on avoiding potential lawsuits, as prison legal scholars Malcolm Feeley and Van Swearingen observe is the case in many, if not most, penal institutions in the United States.[6]

But cutting costs appears to have been a main, if not the most important, motive behind hiring Naphcare to take over health care in all of the state's prisons. One of the governor's attorneys stated to Crowder, "You're negotiating for the best price—there's always a lower number."[7] In a further damning revelation, Crowder discovered that this attorney had a background in contract law and knew nothing about prison health but was hired by Governor Siegelman anyway. The governor's lawyer told Crowder: "I'm a corporate lawyer and have never worked in any kind of prison health care at all . . . I certainly had no experience in corrections contracts."[8] He told her that, focusing on preventing future lawsuits, he "negotiated a contract with Naph-care for about $29.5 million a year, a figure that gave Alabama the low-est per-prisoner health costs in the country."[9]

Like many other states across the nation, Alabama wanted to have its punitive cake and eat it to. Despite massive increases in the prison population and the growing health epidemics behind bars, the state was committed to achieving its objectives of mass incarceration and "tough" (actually, financially strapped) penal institutions. But to achieve this meant turning a deaf ear and a blind eye to a looming health care disaster behind bars.

SCHR Confronts the Crisis

It was clear to Lipman and Zahren that Naphcare's administration of Limestone's HIV/AIDS health services was in shambles. HIV+ pris-oners were receiving neither adequate preventative nor emergent care. The result was the spread of deadly infections, especially Pneu-mocystis carinii pneumonia (PCP).[10] This infection that had all but been eradicated in the Western world was spreading like wildfire in-side Limestone. Lipman explains:

> They weren't providing the people the medication they needed, and the conditions of the dorm itself were so conducive to causing lots of differ-ent diseases and illnesses that are related to untreated HIV and AIDS. The spiders and the filth, the rain coming in, the lack of air-conditioning in the summer and the lack of heat in the winter [were] causing illnesses to appear. I mean, there are two hundred guys living in this one dorm, and they are closely confined, so it is really easy for a contagious illness to spread among the population.

Lipman describes the first prisoner with PCP that he became aware of as follows:

> He was an amputee, and his prosthesis for his leg no longer fit him prop-erly. He had gained weight, and the prison was refusing to provide him with a refitting, so he was confined to a wheelchair. The dorm itself doesn't have any kind of railing for people who are disabled in the shower

or beds or anything. He was hopping around in the shower and would fall in the shower on numerous occasions. On one occasion, he fell and was injured and was lying in the shower water for thirty minutes until nurses came and were able to assist him. There were no ramps for the wheelchair, to get out of the dorm to go outside, so he was stuck inside these horribly close living quarters, and he contracted PCP. Then four to five others got it, and the most recent person died just before the New Year [2003].

Just when Lipman and Zahren thought they had heard it all, things only seemed to be getting worse. But they pressed on, trying to inform ADOC and Naphcare that the situation was far worse than an insect problem. Letter after letter and phone message after phone message were never answered. When SCHR demanded that prisoner medical records be turned over to Dr. Tabet, ADOC refused. This was the last straw; SCHR filed suit in November 2002. Lipman recounts:

One of the initial problems that we had was that they were putting up as many barriers as they could. We had signed medical releases from the people we talked to, so we could try to get their medical files and have Dr. Tabet look at them. We needed Dr. Tabet to see what was happening and to assess what kind of treatment was going on at the prison. We wrote numerous requests listing the names of clients that we wanted the medical records for. But the Department of Corrections refused to provide us with medical records. It was just an all-out attempt to block us from addressing this situation. I mean, we had the prisoners themselves writing to the prison medical provider and asking for the records to be released to them, and they refused. They said that the prisoners were not privy to their medical records. So that was pretty much that . . . We knew we had a very strong case, so we filed suit.

The Impact of the PLRA

After the suit was filed on behalf of the plaintiff class in 2002, Limestone began to reluctantly turn over records to SCHR's medical expert, Dr. Stephen Tabet. With a leading expert on infectious diseases in penal institutions given access to the all-important medical records of recently deceased HIV+ prisoners, SCHR's hopes for putting an end to needless suffering and death seemed within reach. But for Lipman, it had come far too late. Despite what proved to be a pivotal moment in the litigation, Lipman contends that the PLRA was directly implicated in ADOC's stalling tactics and subsequent prisoner deaths.

It's just really hard now because the law, especially the PLRA, has just put so many restraints on the judges, where the judiciary used to protect people who were poor, who were in prison, who didn't have a voice in the government. For these people, the judiciary was the only branch that could really address poor prisoners' concerns and their problems. The PLRA has restrained them immensely. Now that one forum that prisoners and poor people had is gone. They just don't have the same relief or the same assistance that the judiciary used to provide. That's the tough part: the law is so limited. I mean without the PLRA, we could have gotten our work done much quicker, and we would have the ability to ask for more relief for the clients than we can get now. One of the PLRA's most damaging provisions is that we have to exhaust administrative remedies of the facility. The prisoners have to file grievances and allow the facility itself to make correction, before they are allowed to get into federal court. I mean, it's 2002, and this terrible situation had been going on for years and years, but we had to still wait months while prisoners wrote grievances and raised issues that were happening to them. We saw these forms that said, "I have these boils and need to see a doctor." And nothing happens. But you have to go through that system before you are allowed to go into federal court. During that time, we lost numerous prisoners who died because of the PLRA. These issues should have been in front of the court long ago, but we were forced to wait and watch our clients die.

The Challenges of Litigating on Behalf of HIV+ Prisoners

On November 18, 2002, five HIV+ prisoners (Antonio Leatherwood, Eric Howard, Jerry Sanford, John Levins, and Michael Patrick), represented by SCHR lawyers, filed an action on behalf of all HIV+ prisoners confined at Limestone prison in Harvest, Alabama. Taking on Limestone's poor health care was by no means a new challenge. Since the early 1980s—indeed, from the earliest years of the AIDS epidemic—the ACLU's National Prison Project (NPP) has fought for better care and more humane living conditions for the HIV+ populations at Limestone and at Tutweiler prison (Alabama's women's correctional facility). As a litigation project aimed at impacting prisons nationally, the NPP focused its energies on Alabama in the hope of convincing federal courts to mandate broad systemic changes to the nation's prisons as a whole.[11]

Although the NPP had brought some significant reforms to Alabama's prisons throughout the 1970s and early into the 1980s, the dramatic punitive turn in U.S. crime policy (e.g., mass incarceration) and the steady shift to a judiciary that was far less friendly to prisoners threatened to undermine the ACLU's national prison reform strategy. As prior studies of impact litigation on prison reform, such as that by legal scholar Susan Sturm, reveal, "litigation is an interactive, dynamic process involving judicial officers, litigators, and other public officials, which further complicates the task of determining its impact."[12] The increasingly hands-off approach to prison cases taken by the judiciary had seriously hampered NPP's sweeping reform strategy.

This "toughening" of political and judicial approaches toward prisoner rights and conditions of confinement could have hardly come at a worse time. The HIV epidemic had begun to explode behind bars, and reports of prolonged suffering and high death rates of HIV+ prisoners across the United States had begun to mount. Although the NPP had a remarkable record of successes in convincing progressive judges to order systemic changes to Alabama's notoriously inhumane jails and prisons throughout the sixties and seventies, the new world of antiprisoner rights and a judiciary far more deferential to prison and jail administrators made the prospect of successfully challenging conditions of confining prisoners with HIV and AIDS increasingly more difficult. In the two decades since the epidemic struck in the early 1980s, the ACLU's NPP lawyers aggressively attacked the grossly deficient care and treatment of Limestone's and Tutweiler's HIV+ prison populations. At the center of the ACLU's case was ADOC's continued practice of segregating all HIV+ prisoners from the general population, a practice that denied HIV+ prisoners' access to employment, education, and many other important programs available to the general population. The ACLU believed that the dreadful conditions were directly connected to the veritable disappearing of Alabama's HIV+ prisoner population vis-à-vis the state's aggressive segregation policy.[13]

On two separate occasions, despite being confronted with an imposing record of preventable suffering and deaths, the Eleventh Circuit Court of Appeals upheld as constitutional Alabama's treatment of HIV+ prisoners.[14] By the late 1990s, the judiciary's "hear no evil, see no evil" approach to these cases had catastrophic consequences for HIV+ prisoners in Alabama. Reports of prisoners with AIDS being left untreated and thus condemned to die slow and tortuous deaths began to make their way into the national media (see the introduction to the present study). In 1999, the Eleventh Circuit upheld Alabama's policy in an eight-to-three ruling in *Onishea v. Hopper*. By January 2000, the U.S. Supreme Court denied the ACLU's appeal.[15]

Enter SCHR

For years, prison litigation projects, such as the Atlanta-based SCHR, had implemented what Susan Sturm has called an "implementation model of public interest advocacy" in jail and prison cases.[16] SCHR's focus was on bringing forward cases that were strong on their merits and, most important, that held the potential for rapid change. In the Limestone case, SCHR's first objective was not to challenge the state's segregation policy outright but to compel ADOC to improve conditions of confinement. SCHR decided first to negotiate.

Taking its cues from the activist mediation tactics described in chapter 4, SCHR turned first to a much more aggressively activist approach to advocacy. This approach emphasized a focus on communicating to prison officials the special importance of combating HIV/AIDS behind bars. In situations involving other institutions, activists and prisoners alike had demonstrated to officials their unique expertise and had been given greater access to the system (see chapter 4).[17] Rachel Maddow's insights were, at least at first, very important to SCHR. Describing how the activist approach to prison health advocacy has been successful in the past, Maddow explains the logic behind such an approach.

Except through radical oppositional methods, it has been hard to attract the attention of outsiders to prison conditions and prisoners' rights. Prison health care, like other prison conditions, has been treated as a prison issue, both in terms of who has provided care to prisoners (physicians under the employ of prison officials), and who has responded to prisoners' complaints and calls for reform . . . In much the same way that prisoners are removed from their communities, it seems that prison conditions have been sealed off from other political issues. The HIV/AIDS movement has proved an exception to this dynamic.[18]

From the standpoint of the literal life-and-death stakes of this case, SCHR needed to use the media to make the oppressive conditions of the situation at Limestone as transparent to the general public as possible. They knew that the very legitimacy of the current situation had to be confronted. By attempting to create a "legitimacy imperative"[19] — what sociologists of organizations describe as a powerful, media-driven pressure that competing organizations use to create public attention and increased scrutiny around a particular problem — SCHR tried to cast the Limestone case as more than just another prison horror story. They knew that use of the public domain to challenge the legitimacy of ADOC's actions was vital to its ultimate success.[20] Most important, SCHR wanted immediate care for Limestone's HIV+ population, and a focus on mediation and education seemed a promising means to achieving this vital end.

But during the months leading up to the filing of the lawsuit, ADOC did not indicate to SCHR a willingness to cooperate. Given the building body counts, SCHR's gut reaction was to immediately file a class action lawsuit. Although SCHR attorney Tamara Serwer had success using an activist approach in the Fulton County Jail case (see chapter 2), the prospects of achieving a similar result at Limestone appeared less and less likely. Josh Lipman observes:

I mean, how many times can we try to show them that we want to fix this dangerous situation? How many times do we have to call them? How many letters do we have to write before they understand that this is a huge crisis where many more people will likely lose their lives if something isn't done immediately?

Despite the obvious strength of this case, SCHR decided to hold off on immediately filing suit. As a longtime activist who had developed a close relationship with SCHR lawyers over the years, Rachel Maddow urged them to continue to try to meet with representatives from ADOC and Naphcare, in hope of convincing them that improving conditions and care for HIV+ prisoners was in the interest of all parties.[21] Before I continue with how SCHR's strategy ultimately developed, it is important to discuss in more detail the background and potential for success of Maddow's activist approach to prison health advocacy.

Rachel Maddow's "No Lost Causes"

In 1998, just a few years prior to SCHR's involvement in the Limestone case, longtime advocates Ellen Barry and Angela Davis (see chapter 4) established a committee of former prisoners, activists, academics, and families of prisoners to organize a three-day conference called "Critical Resistance: Beyond the Prison Industrial Complex." Building on Davis's high visibility, the conference drew more than three thousand people from around the world.[22] By and large, members of the conference's organizing committee described the event as a success. Two of the most important accomplishments were the building of regional chapters of the Critical Resistance organization in the United States and the realization that conferencing could once again be a very effective tool for organizing and building momentum. In short, rather than focusing only on the national picture, Critical Resistance provided tools and support to activists struggling for prisoner rights at the local level.

Energized by the Critical Resistance conference, Maddow put her efforts into an issue subsequently addressed in *Leatherwood*: finding a way to demonstrate to prison officials that it was in their and the state's interest to address the pain and suffering of HIV+ prisoners. Drawing on a strategy similar to the one utilized by Ellen Barry's National Roundtable on Women in Prison (see chapter 4), Maddow organized a conference of her own. The early momentum for what would be a remarkably successful event began with an emotional discussion between Maddow and a journalist friend about the Supreme Court's unwillingness to end Alabama's oppressive policy of segregating all HIV+ prisoners from the general population. Maddow describes their decision to draft an initial sign-on letter.

It was 2000, and we just got really mad at the Supreme Court decision not to hear the case. My friend knew Margaret Winter (lead attorney for the NPP), and I knew activist people from all the activism I have done over the years. We decided to do a sign-on letter to all the people we considered to be authorities, advocates, and activists in the country on HIV and prisons. We knew an overwhelming majority would join us in condemning the Supreme Court's decision and the role of the Justice Department in it. So we got a bunch of people to sign on to this letter and just sent it out to the press not knowing what was going to happen . . . It ended up really snowballing in that nobody we invited refused to participate, and most people (medical experts, activists, lawyers) were all legitimately outraged. And we realized there actually was a wellspring of people who were authorities on the subject that were interested in it and cared about it. They were pissed and didn't have any way to express that. There wasn't any sort of national voice to express outrage about this, and the ACLU was party to the suit that the Supreme Court rejected, so they were mad, but that was to be expected. But our goal was to make clear to prison authorities that anybody who knows anything about this issue thinks this is an outrage.

Sensing that organizing a broad-based coalition of doctors, activists, and lawyers could be successful, as it was in the *Shumate* litigation (see chapter 4), Maddow convinced the ACLU's NPP to both fund and cosponsor a conference called "No Lost Causes: An Action Meeting on HIV and Hepatitis in Prison." Maddow describes how the conference provided opportunities to confront segregation of prisoners in Mississippi and Alabama in follow-up meetings.

What was great about the conference was that people did really come from all over the country, including Mississippi and Alabama, which at that point were the last two states that segregated HIV+ prisoners. I really pushed for the idea that it would be called "No Lost Causes." And the meeting was held in June of 2000 and was a huge success. And after that, over the next several months, we would have follow-up meetings in both Mississippi and Alabama in order to persuade them to end their segregation policies.

Before discussing the outcome of the follow-up meetings, it is important to recount in detail the significance of the "No Lost Causes" conference to prisoner rights advocacy more broadly.

"We Are Still Going to Win!"

One of the great legacies of the "No Lost Causes" conference may very well have been a broader recognition by the prison legal community that a shift in strategy was necessary to confront the hostile, post-PLRA universe. Maddow elaborates on how she was able to convince the litigation-centered ACLU to support the event.

> I mean, I think it's really important that the whole reason this mobilization started was because the lawsuit failed at the highest level. It was the stupid Supreme Court decision the Justice Department had something to do with it, but it was that litigation had hit a wall. And it was the bravery of the ACLU National Prison Project to get behind this and fund the conference. The point of the conference was to focus national attention and pressure on these policies. And that it is a totally different thing for a litigation-centered organization not to sue. They decided we are going to focus pressure nationally, put tremendous political pressure on these states. And we are going to help people to organize to change these states' policies.

Maddow believes that the success of the "No Lost Causes" conference demonstrates that a litigation-centered project, such as the ACLU, can play a very meaningful role in the struggle for prisoners' well-being, even in an era hostile to prisoner rights.

> It shows them that they are an organization that's willing to make a necessary adaptation to survive in the post-PLRA universe . . . That's the difference between reformists and revolutionary prison work: you have to be evaluated on whether you are increasing the amount of information and the transparency between prisons and the outside world, because that is the engine that will drive all improvements in all activism. And that's why I really wish we would have already won in Alabama, because I want them to think this is something they can apply to other cases and not something that drags on forever. I know the NPP are getting itchy feet: they want to sue. And I'm like, "No! No! We are still going to win!"

The "No Lost Causes" conference was by all accounts a dramatic success.[23] Not only did it bring national attention to the fact that a broad coalition of health experts, attorneys, activists, and prison officials believed segregating HIV+ prisoners was a failed policy and that the situation was not simply a "prison issue," but the conference produced actual results.

Success in Mississippi

In meetings shortly after the inaugural "No Lost Causes" conference had ended, Mississippi prisons officials agreed to end their state's policy of segregating HIV+ prisoners and to improve care. Maddow's coalition demonstrated to state officials that, as evidenced in the number of lawsuits and preventable medical problems associated with quarantining HIV+ prisoners (see chapter 6), ending segregation policy would result in a more humane approach to care and in significant long-term cost savings to the state. Jackie Walker, a longtime NPP advocate, a member of Maddow's "No Lost Causes" coalition, and an attendee at the follow-up meeting with Mississippi prison officials, explains:

> The "No Lost Causes" coalition presented its recommendations to Mississippi's commissioner of corrections. It became clear to them that this policy was simply not in the best interest of the HIV+ prisoners. We recommended that the state end the segregation policies, and then he signed it. So there you go. It was completely grassroots organized. Activists were pissed off and came together and thought up a strategy and then went in that community and worked on it along with prominent members of that community.[24]

ADOC Refuses to Cooperate

Although Maddow's "No Lost Causes" model was clearly an important influence on how SCHR would approach the Limestone case in the beginning, the lack of cooperation on ADOC's part eventually led them to file suit.[25] One important reason why SCHR filed suit was that grassroots activism on behalf of HIV+ prisoners was less effective in Alabama than in Mississippi. Indeed, Jackie Walker described a far different state of affairs at the follow-up meeting held in Alabama.

> Our mission in Alabama was to get the community organized. And we had two meetings concerning both Limestone and Tutweiler. And that was a really difficult situation, because there is more of an openness in Mississippi and also because there was a mother of a prisoner in the organizing group in Mississippi. Alabama has just been a real challenge. No one wants to step out on this issue. But we were able to get Roberta Hall, a legislator who was very much interested in this issue, on board for a while. We eventually were able to get some prominent folks interested, where they signed on, and we had an official meeting with Alabama's commissioner of corrections. But there was not much of a response from the AIDS activist community—I think because everyone is just so concerned about their funding. So we never were really able to branch out. So it's been hard in Alabama.[26]

Despite the lack of activism in Alabama, SCHR was convinced that the Limestone case was very strong, irrespective of the PLRA. SCHR's primary objective was to convince ADOC that the medical treatment and living conditions of the segregated unit was not only unconstitutional but counterproductive. The state had already paid exorbitant legal fees over the last many years. SCHR wanted to convince ADOC that ending the segregation policy was thus not only in the prison class's obvious interest but in the state of Alabama's financial interests as well.

But it would not be easy for SCHR to achieve its goal. For prisoner class action lawsuits challenging conditions of confinement to prevail, they must reckon with the following provisions of the PLRA:

- Lawsuits concerning prison conditions are barred under the Civil Rights of Institutionalized Persons Act (CRIPA) of 1983 until such administrative remedies as are available are exhausted.
- If a state prison fails to adopt an administrative means for addressing prisoners' grievances about substandard health care or

any other matter, this failure alone "shall not constitute the basis for an action."

- The courts are permitted (if not encouraged) to dismiss any case that is frivolous or malicious or in which the party "fails to state a claim upon which relief can be granted."
- Without a prior showing of physical injury, a prisoner cannot challenge his or her confinement in a jail, prison, or other correctional facility for mental or emotional injury suffered while in custody.

Requiring SCHR lawyers and their clients to exhaust all of Limestone prison's "administrative remedies" was, to understate the matter dramatically, no small hill to climb. Despite a protracted and well-documented history of failures on the part of Limestone and its various private prison health care providers to provide constitutionally acceptable medical care, ADOC met SCHR lawyers and their clients with a chilling silence and indifference for more than two years (from 2000 to 2002), as described earlier in this chapter. However, now that SCHR had persuaded a federal district court judge to hear an incredibly compelling case, there was a chance that the needless suffering and death inside Limestone's segregated HIV dorm might finally come to a halt.

The Fairness Hearing

The day that Limestone's HIV+ prison class had been waiting for was June 2, 2004. Pursuant to the Federal Rules of Civil Procedure, a "fairness hearing" to formally adopt the settlement was held in order to resolve any of the prison class's remaining objections to the agreement reached with prison officials. Such a hearing is presided over by a second judge—in this instance, U.S. magistrate judge John Ott of the U.S. District Court for the Northern District of Alabama, Western Division—and serves as a final arena for resolving any conflicts between the plaintiff and the defendant. Judge Ott's role in the *Leatherwood* hearing was thus to evaluate the constitutional merits of the circumstances that led to the settlement, evaluate the specific obligations that the settlement agreement imposed on ADOC, and decide whether or not the terms of the settlement agreement were to be adopted.

At the hearing, the plaintiffs proposed remedy was straightforward: Limestone would be required to adopt new procedures for providing adequate treatment and humane conditions of confinement that, in Judge Ott's words, "prevent the plaintiff class from enduring needless pain, suffering, and, in some instances, death."[27] In assessing the merits of *Leatherwood*'s claims, Judge Ott turned to two primary sources of data: an independent audit of Limestone's medical treatment, conducted by Jacqueline Moore and Associates on November 8, 2002;[28] and more than two hundred pages of detailed prisoner mortality reviews, conducted by the plaintiff class's expert, Dr. Stephen Tabet, in February 2003 and February 2004. Ott found Dr. Tabet's mortality reviews particularly persuasive.

> Dr. Tabet's deceased HIV prisoner mortality reviews demonstrate that the inadequate medical treatment is unconstitutional. It is evident that lives were lost due to preventable lapses in the medical treatment. Additionally, the evidence demonstrates an absence of efforts to save lives by taking ameliorative actions such as conducting mortality reviews and ascertaining obvious problems in the medical system and then resolving these problems. HIV prisoners died without necessary intervention by the Limestone medical staff or Alabama Department of Corrections.[29]

Before turning to Judge Ott's decision and its aftermath, it is important to take a closer look at the institutional failures that precipitated the deaths of HIV+ prisoners at Limestone prison. The investigation in chapter 6 will seek to shed light on the conditions inside Limestone prison that help to explain the deaths of forty-three prisoners between 1999 and 2003. The task of chapter 6 is thus to take a closer look at the preventable deaths in terms of the more complex institutional arrangements in which they were situated.

Chapter 6 Normalizing Catastrophic Loss of Life

Seeing so many guys were passing away, you talk to them today and tomorrow they going to the IICU and never come back. It had a tremendous effect in a negative way on all of us, because we had no classes or support groups. So it affected a lot of guys in a negative way, where they would fight all the time with the nurses and doctors, you know, and get write-ups—unnecessary write ups-and stuff. We were able to go up and sit with the guys in the Health Care Unit (HCU). And when they were on their last stage, almost about to die, you know, we could go read the Bible, talk to them, try to encourage them to hold on or whatever. But again that didn't last a year; they done away with that program. And now, for the last four or five years, none of our inmates have been able to go up there and take care of these guys when they go up there. So when they go to HCU they just up there.

—WILSON ROGERS, FORMER
LIMESTONE PRISONER[1]

As discussion in the preceding chapters has shown, the privatization of prison health has largely been inadequate in addressing the varied, often complex needs of chronically ill prisoners. At the time leading up to the *Leatherwood* litigation, attorney Josh Lipman and investigator Lisa Zahren, both of the Southern Center for Human Rights (SCHR), described in graphic detail just how compromised the system of health care at Limestone was. But most of the details concerning the prisoners' suffering and deaths came to SCHR in the form of letters and postevent interviews. Indeed, the PLRA had blocked

SCHR from responding to these prisoners' urgent pleas in the time of their most desperate need.

To expand on Lipman and Zahren's accounts, particularly as they pertain to what was happening inside the Health Care Unit (HCU) at Limestone between late 1999 and 2003, I draw on Dr. Stephen Tabet's expert witness report and his mortality reviews conducted in February 2003 and February 2004. Dr. Tabet's report was extensively covered in the media and is widely available online.[2] However, to preserve confidentiality of the deceased, all names and factual details from the report that might compromise confidentiality have here been changed. Likewise changed to protect confidentiality are names of the deceased and family members mentioned in newspaper articles and presented in interviews conducted by *Birmingham News* investigative journalist Carla Crowder, my primary collaborator on this project.

Limits of Dr. Tabet's Report

The popular media have reported on Dr. Tabet's report in extensive detail. However, one of the limitations of this coverage has been its focus on the details of prisoner deaths in the absence of a closer look at the broader institutional failures that precipitated them.[3] Although several articles go further than the "prison horror story" that characterized the reporting of "Thunderdorm" throughout the 1980s and 1990s, they do not investigate, at any length, the dynamics of institutional failure that is captured by Dr. Tabet's report, which is comprised of more than two hundred pages of detailed mortality reviews and personal impressions.

Dr. Tabet's report provides a window into the dynamics of institutional failure that has come to characterize health care in most U.S. penal institutions more broadly. As a kind of ideal type, the Limestone case sheds important light not only on how preventable suffering and death of prisoners with dangerous illnesses are increasingly commonplace in U.S. penal institutions but on how such catastrophes persist at the institutional level (see also appendix B). Yet Dr. Tabet's reviews are limited in terms of what they reveal about other important details that may not have been directly implicated in prisoner deaths. To fill in this gap as much as possible, I draw on interviews that

Carla Crowder conducted with former prisoners and prisoners' family members (see appendix A for more details about research methods).[4] I begin by shedding additional light on why the decision of the Alabama Department of Corrections (ADOC) to hire Naphcare is important for understanding how such catastrophic failures took place.

Naphcare Takes Over

When Naphcare took over the administration of health care at Limestone in early 2000, the segregated HIV unit was in a state of profound crisis. The situation had been bad enough in Dorm 7, the old "Thunderdorm," a notorious facility used for approximately fourteen years—since Daniel Ryan, the first person with HIV to be quarantined at Limestone, was placed there in 1985 (see the introduction to the present study). But the conditions in Dorm 7 paled in comparison to those inside Dorm 16—the new "Thunderdorm"—and the HCU. Dorm 16, with its rat infestations, frigid drafts, and swarming mosquitoes, in many ways rivaled the internationally reviled "tent city" jail of Arizona sheriff Joe Arpaio—called "America's toughest lawman"—in Maricopa County.[5] In addition to serving prisoners deplorable food and forcing them to wear pink underwear, Arpaio's facility is an open-air cluster of tents that exposes the incarcerated to brutally hot temperatures and sandstorms. As Aranda Shorey reported, as temperatures climbed well past one hundred degrees in the summer of 2003, Arpaio chastised prisoners who complained about the heat:

> It is one hundred and twenty degrees in Iraq and our soldiers are living in tents too. But they have to wear full battle gear, and they didn't commit any crimes, so shut your damned mouths![6]

Considering that many of the HIV+ men at Limestone were suffering from serious conditions well before Naphcare arrived, the new "Thunderdorm" had become especially dangerous. In addition to the deplorable conditions inside Dorm 16, it was dangerously separated by at least a mile from the infirmary. Meanwhile, the HCU itself was a dreadfully cramped facility that forced the physician and physician assistants to share tiny examination rooms. Moreover, as described by

Dr. Tabet, the HCU's emergency call buttons appeared to have long been inoperable.[7] With a protracted record of chaos and disorganization revealed in nearly two decades of class action lawsuits on behalf of Limestone's HIV+ population, one might have expected the state to have at least ensured that the new health care provider would have adequate resources, staffing, and mechanisms to ensure oversight. However, as was discussed in chapter 3, broader political and economic developments in the state foreclosed the possibility that things inside the HCU would get any better. Indeed, considering the long-standing legislative refusal to properly fund health care in the state's penal institutions, the medical catastrophes that would ensue became far more predictable.

In addition to the lack of funding to ensure quality of care, there were increasing demands on politicians to be tough on crime, a shrinking social safety net, and antipoor punitive tax laws (see chapter 3). These challenges merged to form the conditions under which medical catastrophes behind bars could occur. When we consider these conditions, it is all too clear how a catastrophic penal institution comes into being. It is the task of this chapter to lay out in detail the way one such especially destructive institution operated. By focusing on Limestone as an ideal type, the broad objective is to shed light on the more general conditions—likely to occur in other U.S. penal institutions—that necessitate the normalization of deviant practices on the part of prison and jail personnel.

Beyond "Evil Leaders"

Governor Siegelman's cost-cutting strategy in Alabama was not the action of an "evil leader" bent on torturing HIV+ prisoners. Rather, the governor's decisions to aggressively play the crime card fit policy expectations in many states of the time. States were expected to ensure that prison and jail costs were cut to the absolute minimum, to hire corporate attorneys to ensure protection from lawsuits, and to employ an openly hostile approach to prisoner rights (see chapter 3). Without having to say it, Dorm 16 sent a message to the HIV+ prison population—one of hopelessness and despair.

Some of the most glaring deficiencies at Limestone are revealed when considering Naphcare's staff. Naphcare was responsible for the health care of the general male and female prison populations, including those with HIV or AIDS, but the provider lacked proper qualifications to treat a population of this size. Shockingly, the company employed only a single physician and a handful of physician assistants and nurses to run the segregated HIV facilities at Limestone.[8] In short, Naphcare's "hyper-cost-efficient" model fit perfectly with the twin cultural mandates of appearing to the public as both "anti-welfare" and "tough on crime."

But such a policy approach has its consequences. While Naphcare's director of medical operations, Dr. Colette Simon, may have genuinely tried to provide quality care to the HIV+ prisoner population (see chapter 1), such aspirations were utterly unrealistic given Naphcare's staff shortages and profound lack of resources. As will be shown in this chapter, even well-intentioned prison guards were hamstrung by a system that, for all intents and purposes, had run off the rails.

Institutional Failure in Action

Turning to an analysis of institutional failure, it is first important to explain how the setting was organized. The main field in which the deaths occurred was the HCU. In many respects, the HCU was organized far more as a disciplinary setting than as a therapeutic one. Naphcare's approach to prisoners with HIV and AIDS follows closely Michel Foucault's insightful observation that disciplinary regimes in response to health epidemics practice "two ways of exercising power over men, of controlling their relations, of separating out their dangerous mixtures."[9] In this instance, the depersonalized unit status of "prisoner" as less than human and the additional stigma of being infected with HIV combined to create a pervasively lethal form of penal discipline.

It is abundantly clear that a repeated emphasis on controlling the body and regulating prisoner movements is especially problematic for critically ill HIV+ prisoners. Nancy Stoller, a leading sociologist of prison health, observes:

The spatial organization and structure of prison reflect management goals in opposition to the putative goals of a committed health care provider. Where humanistic health practice requires acknowledgement of interconnectedness, prisons are based on principles of exclusion, separation, and confinement. Where physicians and nurses provide care and comfort to those in pain and those who are disabled, a prison system demands discipline and the stripping of identity, possessions, affection and touch. And where medicine attempts to provide cure and management of disease the primary goal of 21st Century corrections (despite the implications of training and rehabilitation in the word "correction") is typically detention and punishment.[10]

In the sections that follow, I articulate the forms characterizing the disciplinary organization of the HCU.

HIV/AIDS in a Zone of Lethal Abandonment

Acquired Immune Deficiency Syndrome (AIDS) is the end result of a usually long-term infection with the human immunodeficiency virus (HIV). In the early years of the epidemic, reports of men with a strange condition that did horrible damage to their immune systems were published in the *New England Journal of Medicine.*[11] Only three years later, in 1984, HIV, a virus that rapidly destroys an individual's immune system, was discovered to be the cause of AIDS.

When a person first becomes infected with HIV, his or her T cells—white blood cells needed for the immune system to function properly—experience a dramatic decline. According to most specialists in the field, if HIV is left untreated, an individual's T cells will decrease approximately fifty cells per year. This loss of T cells creates a heightened risk for skin infections—such as rashes, boils caused by bacteria, or herpes infection—as well as other opportunistic diseases. In short, the lower an HIV-infected person's T cell count is, the more severe such infections will likely be.

In the last decade, the development of combination antiretroviral therapy, or "cocktails," has been remarkably effective in stabilizing T cell counts and saving lives.[12] For more than a decade, protease inhibitors—drugs that block the dangerous protease enzyme—have been vitally important in treating HIV-infected prisoners, even those with very low blood cell counts. Specifically, blocking protease prevents HIV from infecting new cells, thus reducing the amount of virus in the blood.

If such treatment is to be successful, medications must be made widely accessible and properly administered by trained medical professionals. In the context of marginalized communities in the Americas and around the world, much has already been written about the failure to achieve these interrelated goals.[13] When considering HIV-infected prisoners, a recent shift in penal priorities—one that emphasizes aggressive incarceration policies—and an increased reliance on cost cutting have resulted in a dramatic upsurge in substandard health care behind bars, especially for prisoners with chronic illnesses (see appendix B).

The failure to provide comprehensive care for such populations has (not surprisingly) had devastating consequences. For those who do not receive a consistent regimen of cocktails and antibiotics, there is a risk of deadly infections, such as Pneumocystis carinii pneumonia (PCP). PCP is deadly in HIV-infected patients and was widespread in the early years of the epidemic. Furthermore, outbreaks of tuberculosis—a potentially deadly bacterial infection that attacks the lungs and can also spread to the kidney, spine, and brain—have been widespread in the nation's overcrowded prisons and jails. The outbreak of tuberculosis in a cramped, poorly ventilated jail or prison is especially dangerous for those who already suffer from chronic illnesses that compromise the immune system, such as HIV/AIDS.

As a segregated facility, Limestone's HCU for HIV+ prisoners is embodied by disciplinary forms that compromise the therapeutic setting; the HCU is transformed into a zone of lethal abandonment. Such a zone emerges despite prisoners' persistent suffering. Overwhelmed by a lack of resources and proper training, medical staff succumb to stigmatizing chronically ill patients as "prisoners." Nancy Stoller explains, "The institutional fear of the prisoner, based on an oppositional system of the oppressor and the oppressed, repeatedly carries such weight that the counter-discourses of medicine that argue for the primacy of care are overwhelmed."[14]

Although some argue that prisoner status—irrespective of chronic illness—forecloses one's entitlement to humane treatment, that rationale begins to crumble at the level of health care delivery for the uninsured, represented disproportionately in impoverished communities and in the nation's jails and prisons. Focusing on what kind of treatment individual prisoners are entitled to—often couched in the language of deterrence (i.e., "prisons need to be inhumane to discourage future crime")—ignores the larger problem of the uninsured more broadly. Although this is a line of argument I take up in more detail in the conclusion to this study, it is important to provide some clarification here.

Drawing on a recent study of America's uninsured by Susan Starr Sered and Rushika Fernandopulle, it becomes clear how myopic individualized rhetoric has become in this age of mass incarceration. Consider one of the authors' most politically active, uninsured respondents, "Sue," an individual who provides insights that Sered and Fernandopulle conclude put their entire project into grim focus.

> When Sue, founder of *Collective Home Care*, told us about her recent heart attack, we asked her, "Aren't you scared to be without insurance, isn't that uncomfortable, don't you feel insecure?" Sue answered slowly, thoughtfully, in words that helped put into focus the sense of unease that had been building for us throughout this project. "I'm scared being in our culture, *we're* all in trouble. It's not 'comfortable' for me to work with people who don't have a living wage and don't have health insurance. That's not 'security'—even if I have insurance for myself."[15]

Sue's response focuses our attention in a more productive and realistic direction for the analysis of broken health care at Limestone prison. Instead of being distracted by a narrow emphasis on individual prisoners and punishment, we must explore these issues for what they more accurately represent: widespread institutional failures.

The Institutional Anatomy of Deadly Discipline Inside the HCU

My analysis of institutional failure inside Limestone's HCU begins with a central question: how were the discourses of medicine and the primacy of care overwhelmed at the operational level of the HCU?

The answer to this question is revealed in Dr. Tabet's mortality reviews. His two-volume document presents a striking account of institutional failure, characterized by prisoner suffering, death, and struggle. Most important, the analysis reveals how institutional failure led medical staff to adapt various deviant protocols for normalizing prisoner deaths. Such normalizing practices are revealed in the circumstances of particular prisoners. Issues surrounding the distribution of medications, prior medical histories, and end-of-life care are revealed to be particularly salient contexts for the normalization of prisoner suffering and deaths at Limestone.

The next several sections of this chapter are intended to demonstrate the primary tactics of "deadly discipline" that the HCU staff employed. My analysis centers on a select few cases from Dr. Tabet's report that elucidate how institutional failure from the top (e.g., Naphcare's lack of adequate resources and qualified staff) played out in the actual deaths of HIV+ prisoners. Such an "institutional anatomy of deadly discipline" is realized in three, often interrelated practices: medical personnel label dying prisoners as "poor historians," "poor compliers with medication," and "DNR." All three of these labels embody a particular set of deviant adaptations to a lack of material and educational resources within the HCU. Such practices are driven by a lack of proper record keeping, the failure to implement adequate strategies for addressing prisoner compliance with medication, and the lack of hospice care. In the sections that follow, I draw on specific cases from Dr. Tabet's mortality reviews and explore each of these dominant forms of lethal discipline.

Poor Historians

A lack of proper record keeping and thus a lack of access to HIV+ prisoners' medical histories results in catastrophic failures to prevent future suffering and death. In short, medical staff is left to make cursory evaluations of dangerously ill prisoners' conditions when the prisoner first arrives to the facility. Such unguided evaluations focus on a prisoner's low body weight, for example, and fail to ascertain the particular needs of prisoners. In many instances, the failure to spot early signs of danger results in serious medical emergencies. Such emergencies could likely have been prevented with a more thorough knowledge of the patient's medical history; steps to prevent catastrophe could have be taken. Instead, the prisoner is designated a "poor historian," a person whose long-neglected illness renders them hopeless for recovery. Moreover, staff often express unrealistic frustrations that such individuals are unable to provide them insights into their prior conditions and medical history. Once this "diagnosis" is assigned, the individual's illness becomes something more akin to a ticking time bomb, rather than an ongoing medical condition to be closely monitored and treated.

Henry Davis

Wilson Rogers, a former Limestone prisoner quoted at the beginning of this chapter, told Carla Crowder: "I knew Henry Davis. He got sick and went to HCU and was never returned."[16] For more than ten years prior to admittance to the HCU, Davis had received multiple antiretroviral medications. For years, he was treated with powerful AIDS cocktails. In this way, Davis was one of the lucky ones: he received state-of-the-art medication. But his condition had advanced, and thus other dangerous signs, such as his dramatically decreased body weight, slipped through the cracks. Like so many of the other men in the HCU, long untreated AIDS wasting sickness had taken a severe toll. Davis was now literally a shadow of his former self. Once an energetic and vibrant young man—ex-prisoners described him as "thirty-two years young"—Davis became so emaciated and weakened by the virus that he could barely muster enough strength to get up each morning.

As the result of a severe fungal brain infection, Davis lapsed into a comatose state. But rather than seeking immediate emergency care for Davis, it appears that medical staff decided to stop all further treatment. Indeed, as Dr. Tabet reports, the last staff member to see Davis at this time recommended only that he be "kept comfortable."[17] In the long term, this decision marked the staff's acceptance of Davis's inevitable death. But it also had catastrophic short-term consequences. In a matter of months, Davis went totally blind. Dr. Tabet reports:

For the next couple of months, the medical records and the nursing notes indicate that the patient continued to decline. At one point, the patient develops blindness.[18]

Davis's long history of psychiatric illness would also begin to takes its toll. In addition to his declining health and blindness, he started hearing voices and requested to be put back on antipsychotic medication. But this request fell on deaf ears. In the remaining weeks of his life, nurses only occasionally documented his vital signs.

Lewis Moss

For Lewis Moss, death occurred not inside the HCU but as a result of a heart attack on Limestone's softball field while umpiring a game. Moss had only been at Limestone a few months prior to his death. Despite a host of health problems, he was well liked by the men and relished his time participating in outdoor activities. Much of the surrounding grounds were a space where prisoners could unwind. Wilson Rogers explains how Moss, who had apparently been suffering chest pains for several days, tragically died on the softball field.

> We loved softball . . . But [Lewis] was an older guy, and he was complaining about chest pains for two or three days. And it flared up on the field, so we all went to the HCU with him, and they sent us back to the dorm and told us to fill out a sick card. So five minutes after getting back to the dorm after talking to the nurses, he had a heart attack and died. So their policy was, "No matter what was going on, an inmate must fill out a sick card," and that means twenty-four hours or forty-eight hours later until . . . before they see you, if then.[19]

The HCU's failure to provide care promptly after a prisoner filled out a sick card meant the end for Moss. Unlike the majority of the other men who died inside Limestone prison, Moss's death was not the result of his HIV infection. But it was no less preventable. Moss was pervasively labeled by medical staff as a "poor historian." Despite his suffering from a long history of hypertension, high cholesterol, seizure disorder, and severe diabetes, these conditions were never adequately addressed. Indeed, medical staff did not know that they existed until it was far too late.

In describing his diabetes, the description "severe" that appeared in Moss's medical records was actually a gross understatement. According to the American Diabetes Association, a person with glucose levels of 126 or higher has diabetes.[20] Moss's glucose levels were an extraordinarily high 698. Moss's hyperglycemia was a clear indication that he had not received insulin or other medications to treat diabetes in a very long time. Indeed, medical records from both Limestone and another facility where he was previously incarcerated revealed no indication that he was ever treated for diabetes. When Moss arrived at Limestone, the only medical illness he had been diagnosed with was HIV infection. His other very serious medical problems were apparently never adequately assessed. Dr. Tabet writes that three weeks after Moss's arrival at Limestone, his diabetes and other serious ailments were simply noted by medical staff.

> Apparently no treatments were ever started: [medical staff] reported that the patient had "high blood pressure." The next line states "Diabetes—no meds." This demonstrates that Naphcare medical staff had not reviewed this patient's chart, much less obtained an adequate medical history.[21]

Lack of coordination between Limestone's medical staff and staff from the state's other penal institutions—those jails or prisons that recently transferred prisoners to Limestone—was commonplace. As an elderly male with many health problems, it is clear that Moss had been stigmatized as a "poor historian." Despite the fact that medical records indicated that he had three results for high blood glucose, he was never started on any medications. What is most distressing about this case is that all the warning signs were clear but left undetected: Moss was dangerously diabetic and hypertensive, but the next time he would be seen by medical personnel was after he had apparently collapsed on the softball field.

Gary Terry

A routine chest X-ray discovered something very ominous for Gary Terry. He had developed cotton-ball-sized lesions on both lung fields. The initial belief was that he may have developed lung cancer. However, Terry was never given a lung tissue diagnosis, a routine procedure that staff easily could have performed. A month went by with no further treatment or evaluation. Finally, Terry was given a CT scan, which revealed that it was likely he had developed lung cancer.

In the remaining weeks of his life, Terry's shortness of breath became dramatically aggravated, and he was placed on oxygen and given medication. These treatments, at least for the short term, appeared to provide him with some relief. But it was far too late. As the following details make painfully clear, a lack of proper assessment and monitoring resulted in another lethal calamity inside the HCU.

Over the next few days, Terry would begin literally to start gasping for air. Fortunately, medical staff responded by placing him on a large amount of oxygen, at four liters per minute. All nurses were instructed by Dr. Simon to closely monitor Terry's oxygen saturation level, and if it became less than 80 percent, they were to rush him to an outside hospital emergency room. By 8:30 the following morning, Terry's shortness of breath began to intensify, as he was found by nurses sitting on the side of his bed using his rib muscles to breathe, a kind of breathing common for those with severe emphysema. Another ominous sign became clear to medical staff: Terry's skin color had begun to turn ashen.

One-half hour later, Terry's saturation level began to decrease precipitously, to a dangerously low 74 percent, with a very high pulse rate of 144. Terry had begun to panic. It was then decided by nursing staff that he would have to be transferred to a local hospital emergency room. By this time, Terry's oxygen saturation dropped even lower—to a dangerously low 69 percent.

A little more than an hour later, a nurse's note in the chart describes Terry's transfer to an ADOC vehicle as quite smooth. But this observation was not supported in a sworn statement given by a correctional officer who accompanied Terry.

> I saw the patient get out of bed one time to utilize the toilet. He appeared to be weak with labored breathing at that time. Inmate Terry had a [very low] oxygen [rate]. I stated to the nurse, if Inmate Terry is that bad, shouldn't he be transported in an ambulance.[22]

The nurse declined the officer's request, stating, "He'll be fine!"[23] However, as his statement makes clear, the officer was not persuaded.

> I stated to the nurse that the two officers transporting Inmate Terry do not have medical training to be able to transport an inmate with the problem that Inmate Terry was having. The nurse stated, "He'll be fine. I'll put some oxygen in the vehicle with him and let him roll. He will be fine."[24]

The officer relented and was instructed to drive Terry a full two hours to Birmingham. Officers began the transport and quickly noted that Terry's eyes had fully rolled back into his head. The officers immediately stopped at a store to ask for directions to the nearest hospital. But by this time, Terry had lapsed into full respiratory arrest and was in desperate need of CPR.

The officers were able to get Terry to nearby Woodland hospital, but it was already far too late. Approximately thirty minutes after arriving at Woodland, he went into cardiopulmonary arrest. The nurses attempted CPR. "Even though the staff at the Woodland Medical Center made a valiant effort, the patient died soon thereafter."[25]

Of all the deaths considered in the mortality reviews, Terry's death elicited perhaps the most outrage from Dr. Tabet.

> This is a clear example of the grossest neglect and inappropriate care provided to this patient. The nursing staff should have recognized that the patient should be transferred emergently in an ambulance with trained paramedics to the nearest hospital. He should not have been transported to a hospital as distant as one in Birmingham. This death could have been avoided. This case demonstrates the lack of even a minimal level of medical care and the substandard nursing care at the Limestone Correctional Facility.[26]

Yet when one considers the culture of operational failure that had long pervaded the HCU, Terry's death fit an amoral institutional logic. For one thing, Terry had already been labeled by medical staff as a "poor historian." He had long suffered from both AIDS and a serious form of lung cancer that doubtless caught the ill-prepared staff off guard. The failure to have even remotely adequate monitoring procedures in place resulted once again in a chaotic emergency. Once the situation began to spiral out of control, these failures became most apparent: for the grossly understaffed and unqualified medical staff, the decision to have a literally suffocating prisoner transferred to a hospital two hours away was an extreme but disturbingly normal response. In all likelihood, the nurse had no understanding of just how dangerous the situation had become.

Deadly "surprises" had become so commonplace inside the HCU that it is likely that the nurse's decision to "Let him roll" was not a malicious attempt to injure Terry but a disturbingly routine response by an uninformed staff member. Indeed, without any procedures in place for evaluating just how serious Terry's condition had become, medical staff were responding to the situation as if it had no connection to any previous medical history—indeed, as if taken totally by surprise. To "let him roll" in an ADOC vehicle with a tank of oxygen, was, in the eyes of the staff, the most reasonable course of action.

It is revealing how the institutional failures precipitating Terry's death forced a prison guard to play a role that he was utterly unqualified to play. Despite the courageous attempt by this guard to save Terry's life, the guard was put into a situation that, unbeknownst to him, was set up for catastrophic failure. By going against the orders of medical staff, the guard likely risked his job to save a dying prisoner's life. But to repeat a common refrain in Dr. Tabet's report, it was already too late.

Poor Compliers

Throughout Dr. Tabet's evaluation of the death summaries, several prisoners are described by staff as "having poor compliance with medications." On the one hand, it is possible that some of these prisoners did in fact harbor mistrust toward vitally important medications and flat out refused to take them. But such refusal is not an acceptable basis for care providers to stop all treatment. To the contrary, as Rachel Maddow's research demonstrates, with intensive education and support, even the most noncompliant HIV+ prisoners may agree to treatment.

One of the main institutional challenges to treating noncompliance inside the HCU was a lack of properly trained medical staff, including the use of a single physician to manage health problems

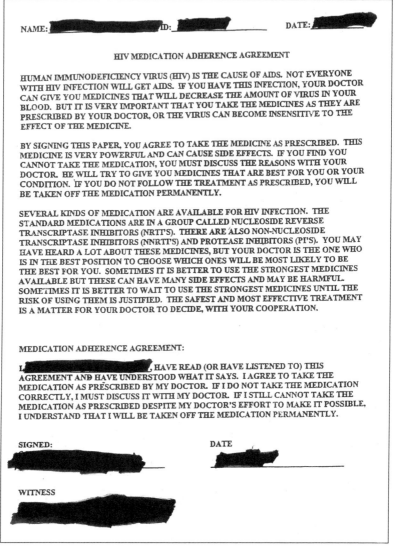

NAME: ███████████ ID: ████████ DATE: ████████

HIV MEDICATION ADHERENCE AGREEMENT

HUMAN IMMUNODEFICIENCY VIRUS (HIV) IS THE CAUSE OF AIDS. NOT EVERYONE WITH HIV INFECTION WILL GET AIDS. IF YOU HAVE THIS INFECTION, YOUR DOCTOR CAN GIVE YOU MEDICINES THAT WILL DECREASE THE AMOUNT OF VIRUS IN YOUR BLOOD. BUT IT IS VERY IMPORTANT THAT YOU TAKE THE MEDICINES AS THEY ARE PRESCRIBED BY YOUR DOCTOR, OR THE VIRUS CAN BECOME INSENSITIVE TO THE EFFECT OF THE MEDICINE.

BY SIGNING THIS PAPER, YOU AGREE TO TAKE THE MEDICINE AS PRESCRIBED. THIS MEDICINE IS VERY POWERFUL AND CAN CAUSE SIDE EFFECTS. IF YOU FIND YOU CANNOT TAKE THE MEDICATION, YOU MUST DISCUSS THE REASONS WITH YOUR DOCTOR. HE WILL TRY TO GIVE YOU MEDICINES THAT ARE BEST FOR YOU OR YOUR CONDITION. IF YOU DO NOT FOLLOW THE TREATMENT AS PRESCRIBED, YOU WILL BE TAKEN OFF THE MEDICATION PERMANENTLY.

SEVERAL KINDS OF MEDICATION ARE AVAILABLE FOR HIV INFECTION. THE STANDARD MEDICATIONS ARE IN A GROUP CALLED NUCLEOSIDE REVERSE TRANSCRIPTASE INHIBITORS (NRTI'S). THERE ARE ALSO NON-NUCLEOSIDE TRANSCRIPTASE INHIBITORS (NNRTI'S) AND PROTEASE INHIBITORS (PI'S). YOU MAY HAVE HEARD A LOT ABOUT THESE MEDICINES, BUT YOUR DOCTOR IS THE ONE WHO IS IN THE BEST POSITION TO CHOOSE WHICH ONES WILL BE MOST LIKELY TO BE THE BEST FOR YOU. SOMETIMES IT IS BETTER TO USE THE STRONGEST MEDICINES AVAILABLE BUT THESE CAN HAVE MANY SIDE EFFECTS AND MAY BE HARMFUL. SOMETIMES IT IS BETTER TO WAIT TO USE THE STRONGEST MEDICINES UNTIL THE RISK OF USING THEM IS JUSTIFIED. THE SAFEST AND MOST EFFECTIVE TREATMENT IS A MATTER FOR YOUR DOCTOR TO DECIDE, WITH YOUR COOPERATION.

MEDICATION ADHERENCE AGREEMENT:

I, ███████████████████, HAVE READ (OR HAVE LISTENED TO) THIS AGREEMENT AND HAVE UNDERSTOOD WHAT IT SAYS. I AGREE TO TAKE THE MEDICATION AS PRESCRIBED BY MY DOCTOR. IF I DO NOT TAKE THE MEDICATION CORRECTLY, I MUST DISCUSS IT WITH MY DOCTOR. IF I STILL CANNOT TAKE THE MEDICATION AS PRESCRIBED DESPITE MY DOCTOR'S EFFORT TO MAKE IT POSSIBLE, I UNDERSTAND THAT I WILL BE TAKEN OFF THE MEDICATION PERMANENTLY.

SIGNED: ████████████████████ DATE ████████████

WITNESS ████████████████████

Fig. 1. HIV Medication Adherence Agreement used at Limestone Prison

among Limestone's entire prison population. Such gross staff shortages led to desperate measures that, in effect, redefined the way poor compliance was addressed; it had become transformed into something that could be used as a form of dangerous prisoner discipline. Instead of taking an aggressive, proactive approach to treating dying patients, it appears that medical staff focused on ensuring that the prisoners were informed of their rights to refuse treatment with minimal follow-up. Indeed, as the use of an HIV Medication Adherence Agreement (see fig. 1) makes abundantly clear, personnel were able, via a banal institutional protocol, to normalize needless suffering and death as a rational choice on the part of the prisoner. The chilling language of the agreement form makes the situation abundantly clear: "If you do not follow the treatment as prescribed, you will be taken off the medication permanently."

Typically, the label "poor complier" resulted in follow-up care, but only at a time when it was far too late. Indeed, the pattern usually followed three interrelated steps: (1) a prisoner signed the HIV Medication Adherence Agreement; (2) the prisoner was documented as a noncomplier in violation of the agreement and was not seen by medical personnel again for many weeks and sometime months; and (3) the prisoner was finally seen by medical staff, but only after the situation had evolved into a dangerous emergency.

Allen Ralston

Wilson Rogers knew Allen Ralston well and describes how his health took a turn for the worst.

> He was a quiet guy. He was very active before he got sick. He liked playing volleyball with us. And his illness just took a toll on him all of a sudden. Actually, he had made parole two weeks prior to getting sick, but he ended up dying at HCU before he was released. And that happened a lot back then. When guys did make parole or whatever, they would always get sick and not make it out.

Running a scorching fever of 104 Fahrenheit, Ralston was rushed from Dorm 16's inpatient unit to Limestone's HCU. Ralston's final resting place was this habitually understaffed, cramped, poorly ventilated facility known by the men as simply "The HCU."

Several months later, Ralston was diagnosed with PCP and placed on oral antibiotics by Dr. Simon. But the fevers would not go away. Even after he was diagnosed, Ralston continued to shiver uncontrollably, literally convulsing through the night without sleep. While some antibiotics are incredibly effective for treating PCP, in this case, they were prescribed simply too late. The *Pneumocystis carinii* organism had already developed into a deadly pneumonia. Indeed, when the physician had discovered it, Ralston's T cell count was already at an extraordinarily low twenty-five, and his viral load was a skyrocketing 295,000.[27]

In the coming months, words uttered by an HCU nurse—"poor compliance with antiretroviral therapy"—would come to mean the end for Ralston. In the chaotic atmosphere of an understaffed, disorganized system of medical care delivery, Naphcare's staff turned often to desperate measures, including one of several forms of deviance from acceptable medical practices: what can best be characterized as "lethal discipline." In Ralston's case, the phrase "poor compliance with antiretroviral therapy" served as code for "stop all treatment." Ralston's identity as poor complier (prisoner) trumped any recognition of Ralston as gravely ill (patient). By viewing Ralston as prisoner as opposed to patient, the failure to provide adequate treatment and care was normalized by medical staff as the prisoner's fault. "Lack of cooperation" with medical staff meant, in turn, a lack of adequate care.

The lack of adequate care became manifest as exclusion, separation, and confinement. Ralston was literally trapped by the preexisting surroundings (the segregated HCU as both a form of separation and confinement), by his inability to move, and ultimately by the medical staff's failure to monitor him. This transformation of the therapeutic space into a lethal zone of abandonment is cogently explained by Nancy Stoller: "Since all places are created and experienced by active human engagement, it is the prison as experienced by the prisoner seeking care that shows us the meaning of moving from one's location where illness is identified to the location where one receives care."[28] In Ralston's case, it was the utter lack of movement that resulted in a denial of care.

Ralston's turn for the worse came when he was not prescribed adequate antibiotics in a timely fashion. To rationalize this egregious lapse in care, medical staff blamed Ralston for his worsening condition. Despite the fact that, in the final year of his life, he was physically incapable of standing in the pill line to receive his medications, Ralston, as a "poor complier," went without treatment. Regardless of the fact that he received inadequate nutrition—a second failure that caused Ralston to literally waste away from AIDS—no action was ever taken by medical staff to rectify what collectively had spiraled into a deadly situation.

If the situation inside the HCU was set up for failure, it is not surprising that medical staff—under orders of their superiors, as an investigative report of the governor and ADOC medical officials would subsequently reveal[29]—focused on meeting minimal standards of care that were protected from legal liability. Documenting Ralston's "poor compliance" thus trumped the need to ensure that Ralston would be treated. Dr. Tabet reports:

> The LPN goes on to list that two of the medications [Ralston] is "34% compliant with" and one of his medications he is "52% compliant with." Unfortunately, there was no discussion with the patient as to why he was not being compliant. He was not asked if he was having any side effects. He was not educated on the importance of adherence. Given the patient's advanced illness, it was unclear whether the patient was even capable of standing in the pill line to obtain his medications.[30]

In the final weeks, Wilson Rogers followed the lead of other healthier HIV+ prisoners before him. He refused to allow Ralston to die alone.

> I was able to go up and sit with him. And when he was almost about to die, you know, I read the Bible to him, talked to him, and tried to encourage him to hold on. I would make sure he ate and drank a lot of fluids, and I changed his linen. I would feed him and talk to him and read to him and stuff like that.

Darrel Simms

Darrel Simms was another prisoner labeled by medical personnel as a "poor complier." But unbeknownst to staff, his severe mental illness had compromised Simms's ability to make a rational judgment regarding his care. Why the staff failed to evaluate Simms properly was crystal clear: Limestone's medical staff was not trained to provide mental health care.[31] For four years, Simms was on very powerful antipsychotic medications, including thioridazine, a drug used to treat patients with disorganized, psychotic thinking and hallucinations or delusions. Yet never once during his stay at Limestone was Simms given a psychiatric evaluation.

The failure to monitor Simms's mental illness was especially dangerous considering his rapidly declining health. In addition to being positive for HIV and having a very low T cell count (less than fifty), Simms had presumptive toxoplasmosis of the brain. A condition not uncommon in people with extremely compromised immune systems, toxoplasmosis is caused by a deadly parasite and, when left untreated, can lead to abscesses, inflammation of the brain, and eventually death.

If Simms was suffering from mental illnesses and a dangerous brain disease, it is not surprising that he was labeled as having a long history of noncompliance with medications. Dr. Tabet explains:

> A note in the chart is representative of the patient's history. It states "noncompliance with Septra"[32] and states he did not need Septra. This medical advice was made when the patient had a high viral load. Septra was needed to prevent Pneumocystis carinii pneumonia (PCP). "He stated he understood and he would not take it because he did not need it" . . . "he understood and will 'pass again.'" From this note, the physician is unsure of whether the patient understands the medical advice being provided or whether the patient had confidentiality concerns or other issues.[33]

As Dr. Tabet's observations make clear, the phrase "pass again" was more than code for a patient's noncompliance; in this instance, it was a de facto death sentence. Despite being obviously incapable of making such complex, life-threatening decisions, Simms was allowed by the medical staff to deteriorate. No record of his autopsy was ever made.

William Watson

According to Wilson Rogers, William Watson was "put in lockup" and died there, because they "kept him there forever." The lockup is an additional, obviously aggressive form of spatial isolation, a segregated cell within the already segregated confines of the HCU. Rogers described it to Carla Crowder as particularly dreadful.

I've been in there. It's a very, very small, tiny cell where you only have enough room basically to turn around in, with a window that stays closed, with a trap door, and they open it just to serve you your tray. You come out for thirty minutes, if at all, a day, and you shower every other day. They take your mattresses. You get no sweets or desserts, nothing like that, and you're in there alone . . . They take your mattress away in the morning at 4:30 a.m. and give it back that evening at 5, so you're on a metal bunk or the hard concrete floor.

The lockup unit prevented Rogers or any other prisoner from making contact with Watson. But fellow prisoners would still try to offer words of encouragement—even though, apparently, Watson was kept in lockup beyond ninety days, contrary to the guards' promises. Rogers explains:

We would be able to go outside the lockup window and yell and talk to him, try to encourage him to hold on. And when we did talk to the captains and lieutenant, they would tell us that they were going to let him out. But they gave him false hope that they were going to . . . Ninety days would pass and they never let him out. So that worried him. He kind of worried himself to death, and with this kind of problem . . . I mean, you don't need to be stressing and worrying when you're already dying.

The lockup obviously took a heavy toll on Watson's health. But his medical records reveal a very long history of serious psychological problems; suicidal behavior was documented extensively by the medical staff. According to records, Watson was first put in lockup after trying to start fires inside the HCU. Despite his extremely low T cell count, Watson was locked down in "the hole" for an undisclosed length of time. Dr. Tabet summarizes the situation in the months prior to Watson's death.

The patient apparently died of Pneumocystis carinii pneumonia with possible secondary bacterial pneumonia, although medical records from the Huntsville Hospital are unavailable. The patient went into respiratory distress approximately five days prior to his death and was transferred to the hospital. He had a very low T cell count of 15. The patient's

chart is riddled with notes of his refusing blood draws and refusing medications throughout almost his entire incarceration . . . There is a cursory
psychological evaluation which states that the patient has a personality
disorder . . . However, one can review these medical records and not find
any in-depth psychiatric or psychological assessment. This is appalling.[34]

As a "noncomplier," Watson was denied treatment. He continued
to experience dizziness and compulsive vomiting. But he would be
left in lockup until it was too late. Watson's untreated PCP led to severe respiratory distress. With a T cell count of fifteen, Watson was
then transferred to Huntsville Hospital, where he died five days later.
In the months after Watson's death, Rogers and other prisoners were
able to convince the warden to improve the conditions of lockup for
HIV+ prisoners. Rogers explains:

> We wrote on that, and they stopped it. And as a result, they give them the
> sweets, they exercise them regularly, and now they do have a mattress all
> day. This guy had mental issues, and he wasn't getting any kind of mental
> health programs or classes, wasn't seeing a psychiatrist and all that. And
> he lost so much weight in there. He wouldn't eat . . . and when he would,
> it wouldn't do any good, because of the diarrhea and everything. And
> they wouldn't let him out; they just kept him there.

"Do Not Resuscitate"

*The goal of hospice care is to improve the quality of a patient's last days by offering comfort and
dignity. Hospice care is provided by a team-oriented group of specially trained professionals, volunteers and family members. Hospice addresses all symptoms of a disease, with a special emphasis on controlling a patient's pain and discomfort. Hospice deals with the emotional, social and
spiritual impact of the disease on the patient and the patient's family and friends. Hospice offers
a variety of bereavement and counseling services to families before and after a patient's death.*

—STATEMENT OF THE AMERICAN
HOSPICE FOUNDATION

A third form of lethal discipline employed by staff at Limestone was
the final transformation of a dying prisoner to DNR status. By contrast to the DNR order that a critically ill patient signs (often with

support of family members) or that is issued by a physician when, as George Smith notes, "there are no demonstrable benefits to a medical intervention that maintains an expiring patient other than the act of survival itself,"[35] the label "DNR" as applied at Limestone became another lethal method for organizing particular prisoners confined to the hopeless culture of the HCU. In short, in the context of Limestone's institutional chaos, the label "DNR" did not indicate a patient acting on his rights but, rather, defined a prisoner category that took on a decidedly different meaning. Like "poor compliers" and "poor historians," prisoners labeled as "DNRs" signed orders as a kind of desperate act of last resort. The signing of such forms ensured that the termination of further care was officially "determined" by the prisoner. The following cases demonstrate how the label "DNR" came to constitute a final form of lethal discipline inside the HCU.

Bobby Reid

Not until the last year of his life was Bobby Reid even diagnosed with multiple myeloma, a cancer of the bone marrow's plasma cells. But the signs of this infection were ever present. Records document that Reid had a blood test indicating abnormally high protein values, and other serious secondary conditions common among those with advanced multiple myeloma had plagued him. In the months prior to the blood test, he experienced kidney failure, AIDS wasting, and decreased mental status. These serious health problems were never adequately assessed by medical staff. Dr. Tabet reports that despite Reid's serious condition, he never received regular blood tests.

> The patient was lost in the medical system and a follow-up was not conducted, or he received no further evaluation for this problem. In fact, the next blood draw was not until approximately five months later . . . The patient's blood draw showed critical laboratory values but were not co-signed until four days later by the attending physician.[36]

Reid's condition was not considered an emergency until he was transferred to Huntsville Hospital. There, Reid was diagnosed with very advanced multiple myeloma. A doctor apparently consulted with Reid's family about end-of-life care. Dr. Tabet reports, "After dis-

INMATE VOLUNTEERS NEEDED

LIMESTONE'S FIRST HOSPICE PRISON PROGRAM

Hospice is a unique program that offers End-of –Life Care for those patients who have a terminal illness where cure is no longer possible.

Hospice addresses the patients' needs holistically with emphasis on physical, social, spiritual and emotional suffering, keeping the patient as comfortable as possible and to allow the patient to have quality of life and a death with dignity.

Volunteers are an essential part of the program. Opportunities include: being a supportive friend/companion - talking with patients - reading - writing letters - assisting with personal care such as bathing and feeding a patient - running errands. The list goes on...offering administrative support for the program such as talking to an inmate group about the Hospice program, etc.....
It may be sitting quietly with a patient during the dying process so he doesn't die alone.
You may have other gifts and talents to offer that have not been mentioned – let us know what those are.

Prospective Volunteers must complete an application and meet the following criteria:
- A minimum of one year left on sentence
- No serious disciplinary reports during the past year
- No positive drug reports whether through the Disciplinary Board or through the courts within the last five years
- No suicide attempts within the last five years
- No documented history of high risk sexual behavior within the last five years
- Medium or Minimum security
- Prior child sexual abuse convictions will be reviewed on a case by case basis
- All volunteers will go through a health screening

All Volunteers will go through a 30-40 hour extensive training program.

If you are interested in becoming a Hospice Volunteer you may pick up an application in the Chapel. After completing the application please return it to the Chapel for processing. Applicants will be notified in writing after evaluations are complete regarding acceptance/denial into the program.
Deadline for submitting applications is November 20th.

Fig. 2. Flier soliciting inmate volunteers for Limestone's hospice program

cussing the situation with the family and the patient on at least three different occasions, the family decided to defer aggressive treatment."[37] Three days later, upon his return to Limestone, Reid was placed on both DNR and "do not attempt aggressive therapy" status. Dr. Tabet noted that during Reid's reintake examination, medical staff recommended "hospice care by fellow inmate and friend."[38] Indeed, it is a clear demonstration of cost cutting in the extreme that despite the obvious awesome responsibilities and specialized training that hospice work entails, such work had become transformed inside the HCU into "just another opportunity to volunteer." As a flier posted in the HIV dorm to solicit inmate volunteers for "Limestone's first hospice prison program" made abundantly clear, "hospice" could mean just about anything, as "the list goes on" (see fig. 2).

In his final days of life, prisoner hospice volunteers were allowed to keep Reid company, but no palliative care was employed to make him more comfortable. It is also clear that no "team-oriented group of specially trained professionals, volunteers and family members"—as generally recommended by the American Hospice Foundation[39]—was ever brought in for emotional support or to monitor any additional pain and discomfort he might experience. In fact, within weeks, the utter lack of hospice care and monitoring of Reid's condition resulted in a very clear indicator of patient neglect inside the zone of lethal abandonment: in the weeks prior to death, Reid had developed a severe bedsore on his rear end.

Ward Anderson

In the final months of his life, Ward Anderson suffered from multiple afflictions, including AIDS dementia, liver dysfunction, and other serious medical problems. When Anderson arrived at Limestone prison, a blood draw revealed that his T cell count was extraordinarily low and that his viral load was dangerously high. It is unclear why Anderson refused antiretrovirals in the coming months, but the HCU staff made no attempt to follow up on this dangerous situation: Anderson simply went without this vital medication.

Anderson agreed to start medication, for reasons never assessed in the physician's notes. The only thing that is clear is that he never made it to the pill line. Like so many others who died between 1999 and 2003, Anderson's inability to negotiate the spatial arrangement of disciplinary "care"—in this instance, the distance from the HCU to the pill line—left him to die in a zone of lethal abandonment.

In the remaining months of his life, medical staff reportedly consulted with Anderson about DNR issues. But Anderson was unsure about these issues at the time of their initial discussion. Dr. Tabet reports, "The patient just wanted to think about it at that point, and specifically did not want to be placed on Do Not Attempt to Resuscitate (DNAR) status."[40] Having gone two full months without any therapy, Anderson was diagnosed with AIDS wasting syndrome. However, he was not started on any oral supplementation or any medications to increase lean muscle mass.

Two months passed before Anderson was seen by medical staff again. When he was finally seen, Anderson was started on nutritional supplementation. Specifically, he was described as "an emaciated male, looking pale and weak." Once again, the decision to be placed on DNR status was discussed with Anderson, but he continued to refuse. In the remaining months, Anderson's health declined. He received very minimal nursing and no hospice care. Contrary to his wishes not to have DNR status, CPR was not attempted at the time of his death.

Creating Alternative Spaces of Care

In her insightful study "Space, Place, and Movement as Aspects of Health Care in Three Women's Prisons," Nancy Stoller argues that HIV+ prisoners confined to substandard prison health care units may attempt to take control of their own care. Commenting on one of the prisoners featured in her study, Luisa Montalvo, Stoller observes, "In Luisa's story, her roommates' help and their determined resistance to the routines that led to her death create embryonic spaces of representation."[41] Despite the isolating confines of the HCU and its attendant zone of lethal abandonment, HIV+ prisoners at Limestone also found ways to resist routines and create new spaces of care. Interviews with ex-prisoners and family members of the deceased reveal that acts for resisting routines and creating alternative spaces involved intimate relationships and the support of family members.

"I'll Never Forget Him"

Thomas Adams, like so many of the men who perished in the HCU before him, progressively deteriorated over many months and subsequently died—"most likely from liver failure, renal failure, and an overwhelming infection."[42] His lover, ex-prisoner Michael Ramsey, described to Carla Crowder how the intimate relationship they maintained provided him with incredible strength to endure life inside Dorm 16.

> I think about him today. I'll never forget him. I know how he looks right now, invisible. I can just sit here and go all the way back and know how he looked. But I know the good things we did. We had some little arguments and fussing, but we never would fight. So we were real tight, real close.

Ramsey went on to describe how Adams protected him upon his arrival to Limestone and how their roles reversed when his partner began to deteriorate.

CROWDER: So it almost seems like your roles were reversed, you know. Like when you first came in there, he helped you out, took care of you.
RAMSEY: Right, 'cause I had nothing, coming in during that time.
CROWDER: And then toward the end, you turned around and were his support.
RAMSEY: Right, exactly . . . I'll never forget him. And can't no other person take the place of him in prison, if I was ever to go back and meet someone. I don't think there's no one on this earth that could take the place of him. My first time in prison, and he had been there like fourteen, fifteen years, until he was experienced, until I knew can't nobody can take the place of him, for me to trust or love or have feelings like I did for him.

"He Was a Human Being and He Did Have People Who Loved Him"

Some of the HCU's most gravely ill prisoners were able to receive visits from caring family members. One such prisoner, Robert Sanders, was often cared for by his sister. Despite Naphcare's reassurances, she was deeply concerned with how her brother was being treated. In fact, she was astonished by his condition. Her description of Sanders is particularly haunting: "He was skeletal, struggling for breath, he hadn't eaten in weeks and blood dripped from his mouth."[43] Sanders's sister describes the last day she saw her brother alive.

The worst feeling in the world was to leave him there. I felt helpless. I felt like there was nothing I could do about it . . . The nurse told me they had done all they could do for him, which is to make him comfortable. He didn't look comfortable to me . . . He was telling me that he was afraid, and I told him to pray, when you get afraid at night just call on the name of Jesus . . . I'm hoping another family member won't have to suffer like that. He was a human being and he did have people who loved him.[44]

Lethal Discipline and the Normalization of Deviance Inside the HCU

There was a pervasive patterning inside the HCU in the final weeks leading up to the deaths of forty-three HIV+ prisoners. The interrelated practices of failed medical record keeping, blaming the patient for their worsening symptoms, and perversely transforming patient end-of-life care into the signing of a de facto death warrant came to characterize operations inside the HCU. As I will show in the conclusion to this study, one doctor's decision to eventually speak out against upper-level corporate prison health managers and the high rate of turnover of Limestone's medical staff elucidates why these lethal practices became normalized.

Beyond the examples from Dr. Tabet's report, all indications are that medical staff knew of the serious problems at Limestone and had likely voiced them to elites on numerous occasions. Indeed, insider accounts of Limestone's broken system of health care had been published in the national media as far back as the early 1990s.[45] Moreover, in the first class action lawsuit against Limestone's flawed treatment of HIV+ prisoners in the late 1980s, numerous examples of similar institutional failures were documented by the ACLU's expert witnesses Dr. Robert Cohen and Dr. Frank Rundle. Like Dr. Tabet more than a decade later, both physicians testified to a kind of routinization of broken health care delivery inside Limestone's segregated HIV ward.[46]

The overriding institutional imperative of cutting costs and protecting against liability trumped the lethal failures of care for the depersonalized and dying prisoners of the HCU. Although medical care personnel rarely went public with their complaints, all indications are that Limestone's medical staff were profoundly dissatisfied with their superiors. Yet it is likely that many medical staff members had become desensitized to the dirty work of managing dying HIV+ prisoners. One need only consider the instance of a nurse ordering a prison guard to let an obviously dying prisoner "roll" to realize that death and suffering had taken on a disturbing banality inside Limestone's HCU. In their insightful study of prisoner medical complaints in one U.S. prison, Michael S. Vaughn and Linda G. Smith observe:

> Socializing correctional medical personnel in an occupational subculture that embraces the custodial/security mission of the institution may diminish their commitment to treatment, healing, and rehabilitation ... In this role conflict, health care personnel may function as "state-supporting victimizers" rather than as "patient-protecting healers."[47]

Nevertheless, turnover among medical staff in America's jails and prisons remains extremely high, suggesting that the role of "state-supporting victimizer" is not one that many feel comfortable playing. High turnover and whistle-blowing (see the conclusion to the present study) occurred among Naphcare medical staff at Limestone, and numerous other states document similar trends.

- A 2004 investigative report of medical care in all New Jersey prisons found that prison medical care under the private contractor Correctional Medical Services "suffered from constant staff turnover and accusations of substandard care."[48]
- One in a series of remarkably detailed investigative reports that the *Columbus Dispatch* conducted in 2003 on Ohio's catastrophic prison system featured reviews of internal memos by prison health care administrators to their superiors at the state's for-profit contractor, Annashae Corporation. One such memo highlighted both an administrator's concerns over potential liability and genuine worry over grossly deficient health care: "We need to do something immediately or we're gonna get sued." Commenting on a doctor who informed an ill prisoner that he "needed to pray to God," the administrator who wrote this memo glibly described such an incident as demonstrating the need for a "more proactive approach to medicine" at the institution.[49]

- In 2001, a nurse at the Massachusetts Correctional Institution–Shirley resigned after blowing the whistle on what she described as the prison's "veil of secrecy" and "sadistic culture." She explained: "Sometimes you come to a moral impasse and you have to act. I just had enough and I quit."[50]
- Deborah Lapham, a former nurse employed by Prison Health Services at Florida's St. Lucie County Jail, sued the company in 2002 under the state's Whistleblower Act. Lapham claimed she was fired in retaliation for reporting that employees destroyed inmates' requests for medical records, refused requests for medical attention, and ridiculed mentally ill inmates. In the same report, a former nurse at Palm Beach County Jail described medication being intentionally withheld from prisoners, especially if they were expensive: "'We have patients that go without their HIV medication for a substantial amount of time,' the nurse said, adding that psychiatric drugs and antibiotics also are withheld."[51]
- Even upper-level private prison health care officials have become whistle-blowers. In a 2005 investigative report of Prison Health Services by the *New York Times,* Barbara Logan, a former senior administrator in Indiana's prison system, described the state's prison pharmacy as "so poorly stocked that nurses often had to run out to CVS to refill routine prescriptions for diabetes and high blood pressure."[52]
- Dr. Roy Kropinak, a former physician at New Mexico's Santa Fe County Detention Center, was fired by Correctional Medical Services after complaining about numerous problems with the company's aggressive cost-cutting tactics. Specifically, Kropinak described to a reporter how the company's staff routinely canceled or delayed his orders for prisoner care and would change his patient orders "without notice, once with near-fatal results."[53]

In this book's conclusion, the whistle-blowing phenomenon among private prison health employees will be an important part of documenting the latest developments in the Limestone case. First, the conclusion turns to Dr. Tabet's final visit to Limestone.

CONCLUSION

On February 23, 2004, approximately four months before Judge Ott would hand down his opinion in the *Leatherwood* fairness hearing, Dr. Stephen Tabet returned for a follow-up evaluation of Limestone's HIV+ prisoners. By this time, the entire population had been moved from Dorm 16 to new living quarters. Units 6A, 6B, 7A, and 7B were, as Dr. Tabet would observe, a marked improvement from the decrepit, insect-filled warehouse.[1] Rather than being packed into one dilapidated facility, the new units housed one or two prisoners per cell.

While the new arrangement appeared to be more conducive to adequate care, there were still many serious problems. For one, the vast majority of the prisoners complained that the cells were cold, especially at night. More distressingly, none of the cells had emergency call buttons. Additionally, Dr. Tabet found that the notorious pill line was still operating at a suboptimal level. Indeed, he discovered that once again, several prisoners were not receiving all of their appropriate medications. Moreover, he reported that the medications continued to be administered improperly.

> The pill line was a disaster. Numerous patients did not have their medications on hand and were told to come back, or were told that they did

not have the medications altogether. Also, as described in the previous visit to Limestone Correctional Facility, many of the medications that are FDA approved to be administered with food, were in fact being administered without food . . . Sometimes the separation of the medications with food is as much as one-and-a-half hours. This leads to excessive side effects, including nausea, vomiting, and diarrhea, and poor medication absorption.[2]

In short, Dr. Tabet found that serious problems remained. Most glaringly, prison officials still had not implemented a formal method for reviewing patient deaths. Dr. Tabet observed:

This is a very disturbing problem that needs to be urgently addressed. All patient deaths need to undergo a full internal and external autopsy, and all deaths need to be reviewed in detail by an outside physician/monitor. In addition, the staff needs to provide more compassionate education to patients before signing "Do Not Resuscitate" orders.[3]

Dr. Tabet's visit also uncovered a new, particularly disturbing revelation. Incredibly, he discovered that Limestone's warden and Naphcare's physician had never once been in contact with one another.

The analogy I would use that exists at Limestone is that the head of the institution (the Warden) has been severed from the body (the Medical Director). Initially, the Medical Director should write detailed monthly reports describing the components of the medical system and ongoing medical activities. This report should be reviewed by an outside, independent monitor. An outside independent monitor should review Naphcare's physician's clinical decisions.[4]

Moreover, the medical staff continued to be dangerously understaffed. Prisoners continued to serve as "runners" for the dying. Nutritional supplementation continued to be administered below minimal requirements. While Dr. Tabet was unable to reassess whether medical emergencies continued to be a problem, a recent prisoner's death only confirmed this to be the case.

The Leatherwood *Settlement and Its Aftermath*

As SCHR finished its investigation, it became clear that Dr. Simon should not be singled out as the "bad apple" to take responsibility for the systemic—indeed, catastrophic—conditions that had characterized the HCU from 1999 to 2003. The very high attrition rate of Naphcare's employees also signaled to SCHR that there was likely a long history of dissatisfaction on the part of staff. SCHR instead locked its sights on Naphcare and the ADOC officials. Concerning the former, Naphcare would eventually be fired by ADOC and replaced by Prison Health Services (PHS). Naphcare's dismissal was but a footnote in the overall, still unfolding drama of *Leatherwood.*

It is important to take a closer look at the settlement agreement. First and foremost, the hearing resulted in the settlement that SCHR had hoped for. The court ordered ADOC to hire a full-time HIV specialist and a coordinator to ensure follow-up care. Moreover, among other important provisions of the settlement, ADOC was ordered to improve staff training, to conduct six day evaluations for all prisoners with HIV and AIDS, and to implement an all-important plan for infection and a formal policy for addressing medical emergencies. Given more than twenty years of unsuccessful litigation against ADOC by the ACLU, this was certainly a major milestone for SCHR. In the face of a protracted history of refusals to do anything, the *Leatherwood* ruling provided the first real hope for Limestone's HIV+ prisoner class.

"No Closer than the Day the Document Was Signed"

Unfortunately, after the *Leatherwood* ruling, the situation was far from over. With the litigation now out of the way and the controversial PHS on board, ADOC decided to ignore many of the crucial specifics included in the settlement agreement. On February 17, 2005, only ten months after federal magistrate judge John Ott certified the order, SCHR filed a second class action lawsuit against ADOC, for failing to comply with the terms of the settlement agreement. As Joshua Lipman stated, "the Alabama Department of Corrections' attempts to provide even a minimal level of acceptable medical care and housing to HIV prisoners at Limestone is appalling."[5] Among other serious problems persisting at Limestone were gaps in medical distribution, persistent delays for routine medical checkups with an HIV specialist, broken windows in the HIV dorms, and continued inadequacies in responses to medical emergencies.

Another important factor after the *Leatherwood* ruling was that members of the medical staff continued to resign. This development elucidates the more complex story of catastrophic penal institutions that I have attempted to tell throughout this study. Institutional crises are complex, unfolding dramas that are not easily cabined by romantic narratives that draw clear lines between heroes and villains. Most striking, when the newly hired replacement for Dr. Simon confronted her superiors at PHS about the serious problems that persisted at Limestone, she was formally reprimanded by her supervisors and shortly thereafter resigned.

Valda Chijide: From Prison Doctor to Whistle-Blower

It is interesting to consider the details leading up to the resignation of Simon's successor, Dr. Valda Chijide. As the result of *Leatherwood,* a medical monitor was now making routine trips to Limestone to evaluate whether or not the stipulations of the settlement agreement were being met. When Dr. Chijide became clearly convinced that they were not, she first made her concerns known to PHS in writing. She did not hear back from her superiors until she was called in and given a formal reprimand. After weeks of a frustrating lack of feedback from PHS, all Dr. Chijide received in return was a sanction. Refusing to remain silent, Dr. Chijide wrote a detailed letter to lawyers from SCHR.

Dr. Chijide informed SCHR how little progress had been made toward the settlement's critical stipulations to improve staff training, prisoner evaluations, and emergency plans; PHS was not responding to her desperate calls to have the continued lapses in care addressed. Indeed, as the weeks ticked by, Dr. Chijide became overwhelmed by the dangerous outgrowths of PHS's lack of an adequate response. Delays and failures to obtain proper medication and the inability to quickly access patients' labs or infirmary reports pushed Dr. Chijide's ethical duties as a physician to the breaking point.

A 2005 investigative report by the *New York Times* entitled "Harsh

Medicine: A Company's Troubled Answer for Prisoners with H.I.V."
provides important insight into the events leading up to Dr. Chijide's
resignation. First and foremost, it is clear that PHS never provided
Dr. Chijide with the additional physicians and trained staff that they
had promised. Like Dr. Simon before her, she thus remained the sole
physician in charge of 230 HIV+ male prisoners as well as the rest of
Limestone's prisoner population of eighteen hundred.

Barely three months into her tenure, Dr. Chijide refused to remain silent any longer and confronted her superiors at PHS. She
heard nothing at first and then was notified that she had been sus-
pended. As the *New York Times* reported, Vada Chijide resigned as
Limestone's HIV specialist shortly thereafter.

> "If you bring up a problem that they don't want to hear about, they will
> attack you," said Dr. Chijide, 45. "I felt better resigning than staying on
> and bending my principles to their principles." A Prison Health
> spokesman said the company "had great expectations" but was informed
> that she had violated company policy, though it would not say how. She
> was put on leave, the company said, and before it could investigate, she
> quit.[6]

Of Dysfunctional Organizational Authority and Whistle-Blowing

In addition to being what the *New York Times* characterized as a "a
rare firsthand account of a doctor in charge of a prison's health care,"[7]
Dr. Chijide's account reveals what sociologists have long observed
about dysfunctional organizational authority and whistle-blowing, as
explained by sociologist Robert Perrucci and colleagues.

> Whistle-blowing, as a single visible act, is the culmination of a series of
> actions and reactions that take place in the course of a professional's rela-
> tionship with an employing organization. Therefore, to understand whis-
> tle-blowing it is necessary to identify specific organizational condi-
> tions—authority structure, lines of communication, opportunities to
> participate in decision-making—that give rise to initial acts of disagree-
> ment with, or concern about, some organizational practice . . . Finally, it
> is essential to place the principal actors in a whistle-blowing incident in a

larger context of economic, political, and professional forces impinging upon the situation.[8]

Considering Dr. Chijide's role within PHS, it is clear that all three of the conditions for what constitutes whistle-blowing were relevant in her case. First, the authority structure of PHS had placed her in an extremely difficult position. While she was the head physician at Limestone, PHS failed to supply her with adequate staff and other promised resources. Dr. Chijide also had no clear line of communication with her superiors at PHS. Her letters were not adequately answered, leaving her and her staff in the dark. Finally, she had no clearly defined role in institutional decision making. While Dr. Chijide recommended that many necessary changes, especially the addition of more qualified staff, had to take place in order for her to provide adequate care, PHS only provided her with one additional nurse.

Silence, Disavowal of Responsibility, and the Normalization of Deviance

How does Dr. Chijide's departure provide further insight into the conditions underlying catastrophic institutional failure at Limestone prison? As shown in chapter 6 of this study, the catastrophic failures at Limestone were driven by the normalization of deviant practices on the part of medical personnel, which was the function of an overburdened, underqualified staff who lacked any clear lines of communication with their supervisors. But the analysis in chapter 6 did not adequately consider the role that institutional elites played. Dr. Chijide's whistle-blowing and PHS's subsequent nonresponses—beyond the company's "great expectations for Dr. Chijide"—help to demonstrate the way senior level officials are able to distance themselves from responsibility.

Consider, for example, the *New York Times*'s failed attempt to obtain an in-person interview with PHS's president.

> The company offered in June to arrange an interview with its president, Trey Hartman, but never made him available, and eventually answered only a small number of questions via e-mail. "P.H.S. continues to provide

evidence-based medical care to the patients of the A.D.O.C. in a timely and professional manner," said Benjamin S. Purser Jr., a spokesman for the company, referring to the Alabama Department of Corrections.[9]

The PHS spokesman's "flexibility narrative" is, as sociologists Susanne Monahan and Beth Quinn demonstrate persuasively in their case study of institutional deviance at Abu Ghraib prison, a potent means for bureaucratic elites to distance (or, in the parlance of neo-organizational sociology, "decouple") themselves from lower-level actors.

> The organization effects a sort of buffering of lower-level workers from the environment by offering sufficient flexibility—in the absence of serious monitoring—to accomplish work. When deviance is detected, however, this buffering (i.e., the distancing) may be employed against these lower-level actors as it is now the organization and its leaders who are protected from blame by the process of decoupling and the scapegoating that ensues. In this is embedded the central dynamic of organizational decoupling: that deviance is normalized as long as it is invisible, and disavowed when it comes to light.[10]

PHS elites satisfied institutional demands (i.e., cost cutting) by distancing the company from incidents that called into question its legitimacy and by finding scapegoats (i.e., Dr. Chijide) for wrongdoing.

It is relatively easy for institutional elites in charge of jail and prison health bureaucracies to disavow themselves from wrongdoing. Why is this especially the case today? First, one must consider the political moment. Prisoners are increasingly dehumanized in public discourse. What happens to "them" is less important than what happens to the overriding mission of protecting the society from crime. The objectives of helping those trapped behind bars with chronic illnesses and preventing future crime are unnecessarily constructed as opposing goals in a kind of perverse zero-sum game. Decades of this dominant ideology have led to an unprecedented explosion in the U.S. prison population and to the attendant need to do punishment on the cheap. The overriding focus on cost cutting in this era of unprecedented growth in jail and prison populations has obscured the consequences—namely, grossly inadequate conditions inside many of America's penal institutions today.

Pervasive Institutional Failures

Beyond Limestone, it is difficult to know just how bad things may be in the nation's other penal institutions. It is clear that institutional failures resulting in the needless loss of life are occurring in jails and prisons from every region of the country (see appendix B). U.S. jail and prison medical bureaucracies are routinely understaffed and underresourced, and clear lines of communication between medical personnel and institutional elites are the exception rather than the rule. We thus may very well be witnessing a disturbing trend toward a broader entrenchment of medical catastrophes in the nation's penal institutions as a perversely secret "part of doing time." It is no overstatement to observe that health care in the nation's jails and prisons is characterized by grossly dysfunctional institutional practices that emphasize cost cutting over care, even if such care results in needless prisoner suffering and preventable deaths and in scapegoating of lower-level personnel by elites. But we just don't know how deep these problems go across the states.

Michael S. Vaughn and Linda G. Smith's five-year case study of one jail under federal consent decree provides some important insight. Investigating ill prisoners' medical records and 103 letters sent to a federal court monitor, Vaughn and Smith discovered "a persistent pattern of medical ill-treatment and torture at the jail, which extended over the entire five-year period."[11] To date, Vaughn and Smith's field study, sociologist Nancy Stoller's research documenting egregiously substandard medical care for HIV+ women prisoners in California (see chapter 4), and the present analysis are the only detailed studies that have been conducted to analyze penal health care failures. Beyond media accounts and investigative reports, we lack the kind of remarkably detailed analysis that Dr. Tabet was able to conduct in Alabama. Such an analysis provides truly unique insights into the contours of preventable prisoner suffering and death that are otherwise kept secret in nearly every other state in the nation.

If one considers the penal system in Wisconsin—one of few states that have made prisoner death summaries public in recent years—we can see institutional failures nearly identical to those that occurred at Limestone. While there was no comprehensive report conducted in Wisconsin by a renowned medical expert, several important findings are revealed by investigative reporters who were given access to the death summaries. In addition to a faulty system of record keeping—described as "scribblings on pieces of paper"—and a lack of effective protocols for preventative care, investigative reporters from the *Milwaukee Journal Sentinel,* Mary Zahn and Jessica McBride, documented how cost cutting in the face of growing overcrowding had become the primary institutional imperative of the Wisconsin Department of Corrections. For example, the investigators discovered that in 1999, Wisconsin's prisons employed only a single nurse for every 140 inmates. In terms of fatalities, there have been 123 prisoner deaths in Wisconsin's prisons in little over a six-year period of time (from 1994 to 2000). One interview that Zahn and McBride conducted with a nurse made clear how the state's emphasis on cost cutting risked even more unnecessary fatalities in the future, as "corrections are spending so much money on building they don't want to spend the extra money on health care."[12]

Assessing Proposals for Reform

One obvious response to the Limestone case and the problem of medical catastrophes behind bars more broadly might be to invest more resources in the quality of penal health care. If health providers were given more money by the state, they could hire more and better-qualified staff to ensure better care. The problem with such a proposal is that it is unrealistic for the vast majority of states—particularly those with high incarceration rates.[13] Because mass incarceration has produced more, not less, of an economic burden on states, the overriding emphasis has been to cut costs.

There is a reason cost cutting is stubbornly attached to prison health: prisoners are not popular among the public and lack any kind of political clout, so all jail and prison programs are likely to remain very vulnerable to budgetary cuts. Moreover, it is unclear that more resources alone would lead to comprehensive reform. Given the entrenched institutional culture of secrecy and the pervasive ideology of discipline and control that characterize penal institutions in the

United States today, one wonders if, even with more funding, chronically ill prisoners would continue to be denied access to the kind of comprehensive care they require.

A second proposal is to reduce incarcerated populations in the United States. While there is some evidence of this occurring in a few American states with historically high incarceration rates, such declines are likely to be very gradual, as attempts at reducing penal populations continue to face serious opposition. One recent study sheds important light on the prospects and challenges of ending mass incarceration policies. In *Downsizing Prisons: How to Reduce Crime and End Mass Incarceration,*[14] Michael Jacobson highlights how three states— California, Connecticut, and Louisiana—are attempting to reduce their prison populations. Following the lead of these states, one might contend that reducing penal populations will free up resources for better prison health care and, as Jacobson rightly argues, for prison expenditures to be redirected to the country's ailing education and health care systems more broadly. For example, between 2001 and 2002, rapid increases in jails and prison expenditures meant deep cuts, upwards of eighty million dollars, in Mississippi's K–12 and state university systems.[15]

As Jacobson counsels, one of most challenging roadblocks to reducing incarcerated populations is the difficult challenge faced by politicians convinced that they must appear "tough on crime," a conundrum I take up in more detail later in this conclusion. The historical record makes another troubling state of affairs clear: corrections officer unions, the privatized prison and prison health industry, "tough on crime" victim rights organizations, and the National Rifle Association (NRA) will fight tooth and nail to prevent any attempts a state makes toward reducing penal populations.[16] In Mississippi, massive prison expansion has resulted in powerful coalitions between private prison contractors, lobbyists, and state and county officials. "The result," Peter Wood and R. Gregory Dunaway report, "has been a financial and political bazaar with prisoners as the prize."[17] Lastly, some politicians, most recently California governor Arnold Schwarzenegger, have found ways around the challenge of appearing soft on crime and facing the backlash of unions: export prisoners— like human waste—to other states.[18]

Creating More Access to Care?

Other proposals for reform might entail the deprivatization of penal health care. While some states use nonprofit prison health care providers, it is not clear that this results in better care. One reason for this is that jail and prison medicine does not attract particularly good personnel, and many of the good people it does draw quit as a result of conflicts of interest with prison officials ordered to cut costs by the state. In a damning investigative report conducted by Andrew Skolnick in the *Journal of the American Medical Association*,[19] private prison health companies were found to actually seek out physicians with records of incompetence and to have persuaded some state boards of medical licensure to grant licenses permitting incompetent doctors to practice in prison settings only.

By contrast, one might take a strong market-centered stand and argue for more corporate influence in penal health care. When considering the growing presence of drug companies in penal institutions, this position is more than a recommendation; it has become a reality. Increasing the availability of low-cost drugs is an important and inescapable role for the industry to play, particularly in an age of complex illnesses—such as HIV/AIDS and hepatitis C—that require an abundance of important treatments, given the ability of the industry to continually upgrade such medications.

There are serious concerns with the growing presence of the pharmaceutical industry in America's penal institutions. From prior research, we know that greater availability does not mean greater access. While this concern does not directly implicate drug companies, it does attest to the uniquely vulnerable position of prisoners. In the recent past, prisoners have been used as guinea pigs in dangerous scientific experiments, such as the horrific studies conducted at Philadelphia's notorious Holmesburg Prison in the 1960s. Allen Hornblum's remarkable book *Acres of Skin: Human Experiments at Holmesburg Prison*[20] documents how thirty-three pharmaceutical companies were permitted to test 153 experimental drugs at this facility. The title of the book comes from the fact that most of the abuses were the result of dermatology experiments conducted on uninformed prisoners paid to test various facial creams, hair lotions, skin moisturizers, suntan products, foot powders, deodorants, detergents, and antirash treatments. In a 1966 newspaper interview, corporate-sponsored physician Albert Kligman, a former professor of dermatology at the University of Pennsylvania, ominously remarked of his experience when entering the prison: "All I saw before me were acres of skin. It was like a farmer seeing a fertile field for the first time."[21]

Since Holmesburg Prison closed in 1977, much stricter regulations have been placed on companies involved in using prisoners in any kind of experimentation, including participation in drug trials. At least in the United States, it is doubtful that another Holmesburg could occur. But in August 2006, a high-level panel of medical advisors recommended loosening regulations on testing pharmaceuticals on prisoners, setting off a firestorm of controversy in the national media.[22] There have also been very recent reports of serious problems associated with prisoner participation in drug trials. Specifically, institutional breakdowns in communication between drug companies sponsoring trials at outside facilities and prison medical care providers can increase the potential for dangerous mistakes in treatment.

Consider a recent investigative report of the prison health care system in Texas by the *Houston Press*. The report revealed persistent conflicts between security and prisoner health. When Texas prisoners who participated in clinical trials at a nearby medical facility returned to prison, their newly obtained medications were "flushed down the toilet" by correctional officers.[23] Additionally, doctors in one prison were found to often cancel the orders of prison physicians in another location. The *Houston Press* report also documents the testimony of a medical expert who, after reviewing hundreds of pages of records, told a federal judge that "orders are overridden by unit clinic clinicians and unit clinical pharmacists, apparently without direct consultation with UTMB [University of Texas Medical Branch] prescribing physicians."[24]

Low Incarceration Rates, Coordinated Health Care Response, and "Geographic Advantage"

There are some success stories found in American states—typically in small ones—that have low incarceration rates. For example, the Rhode Island Department of Corrections has established a strong relationship with the state's public health department, Brown University, and a local hospital. Infectious disease specialists from these institutions provide treatment to Rhode Island's HIV+ prisoners and are able to continue that care after prisoners are released.[25]

Can Rhode Island's system be a model for other states? To answer this question, one must first consider the state's incarceration rate. Despite the fact that Rhode Island is well above the national average in terms of racial disparities in sentencing,[26] Rhode Island had the thirteenth lowest incarceration rate in the country in 2004.[27] Rhode Island also has a protracted history of dangerous overcrowding in its prisons and jails.[28] However, the state has largely stuck to a 1977 agreement that required it to vigilantly ensure better conditions in its penal institutions. One clear indicator of Rhode Island's commitment to follow the agreement is that it became one of the nation's leaders in spending on individual prisoners by 2001.[29] In this way, Rhode Island remains clearly an anomaly in the world of penal health care, especially when one considers states with high incarceration rates.

Secondly, Rhode Island is the smallest U.S. state. This fact has significant implications when considering emergent care for critically ill prisoners. Specifically, there is relative ease of transfer between penal institutions and the state's hospitals in Rhode Island—compared to, say, California, a state whose badly broken penal health care system is currently under federal receivership.[30] Long-distance transfers of critically ill prisoners has resulted in preventable deaths even at California's Vacaville prison, an institution that has by far the most comprehensive health care for HIV+ prisoners in the state.[31] But geographic advantage cannot be seen as a panacea. Indeed, the nation's second smallest state, Delaware, has one of the nation's highest incarceration rates, has severe problems with overcrowding, and has a record of dismal and inhumane health care in its penal institutions. Lacking Rhode Island's willingness to invest significant financial resources, coordination between agencies, outstanding university system of care, and progressive public health department, Delaware's system today stands as nothing short of a human rights catastrophe. A 2005 investigative series by the Wilmington-based *News Journal,* entitled "Delaware's Deadly Prisons,"[32] revealed a host of institutional failures leading to deadly lapses in prisoner health care in the state. Prisoners in the state are not screened for hepatitis C and HIV, the state does not conduct autopsies on prisoners who die in prison or those hospitalized at the time of their death, and no systematic way for assessing prisoner's medical complaints exists in Delaware's penal institutions.

Litigation and Harm Reduction Strategies

Certainly one proposal for future class action litigation is to consider seriously the approach SCHR adopted in the *Leatherwood* case. Despite the PLRA, SCHR prevailed, regardless of how limited the successes ultimately may be. By making information available to the public, SCHR empowered investigative journalists from the *Birmingham News* and the *New York Times* to craft powerful and serious coverage of the Limestone case and shed crucial light on the complex problems of prisoner health care in the United States. SCHR enabled these journalists to write reports that went well beyond the sensationalistic prison horror stories that dominate popular discourse in the United States today.[33]

SCHR's approach to litigation also demonstrates the importance of involving prison health experts, such as Dr. Tabet. By obtaining subpoenas to literally open the black box of jail and prison health bureaucracies, prisoner rights litigators can conduct more systematic documentation of the institutional failures leading to needless suffering and preventable prisoner deaths. It seems logical that making the system more transparent will increase the chances that a comprehensive national response to the crisis will occur. Indeed, with the recent passage by Congress of the Deaths in Custody Reporting Act (DICRA) of 2000, a more complete picture of the problem may well be within the reach of policymakers. However, it is unclear whether such legislation has real teeth or is only a symbolic gesture.[34]

Some direct harm reduction strategies to managing the spread of infectious diseases, such as HIV/AIDS and hepatitis C, can be implemented immediately. Given the urgency of the problem, granting prisoners access to condoms and clean needles is an essential first step. While such harm reduction strategies have been widely adopted in Canadian penal institutions, they continue to receive strong opposition in the United States.[35]

Confronting Catastrophic Penal Institutions

Perhaps the most sweeping proposal for directly reforming the nation's penal health care systems is contained in a recent report by the National Commission on Correctional Health Care (NCCHC). While the report is titled "The Health Status of Soon-to-Be-Released Inmates," it does make several recommendations regarding prison and jail health care more broadly.[36] The NCCHC recommendations involve the need for comprehensive institutional-level changes to penal health care systems, including increased surveillance of prisoner health, the use of nationally accepted evidence-based guidelines that ensure the appropriate uses of resources, improved delivery of prisoner health care, and, among other policy suggestions, the implementation of primary and secondary disease prevention behind bars. The NCCHC even goes as far as to advise Congress to require both the secretary of the U.S. Department of Health and Human Services and the U.S. attorney general to be far more involved in overseeing penal health care in the nation: "A Federal interagency task force, currently established and co-chaired by CDC and NIJ, should report annually to the Secretary and the Attorney General on the status of correctional health care in the Nation and on progress made toward implementing the recommendations included in this report."[37]

The Disease of Mass Incarceration

The NCCHC's calls for comprehensive reform and aggressive federal government oversight are laudable, yet one cannot help but think that reformers might be underestimating two profoundly interconnected shifts of the last three decades: the rise and ubiquity of waste management strategies in the nation's penal institutions and the social and political conditions that produced such a profoundly flawed system of penal health care in the first place. Taken together, then, the greatest challenge we face in a nation obsessed with incarceration is how to control institutional forces that generate fiscal crises, lead political elites to emphasize economics over human rights, and result in the normalization of catastrophic captive bureaucracies that engage in the quiet brutality of needless suffering and preventable deaths. Before I explore this broad statement in more detail, I will draw on recent empirical research that confirms the impact of governing through crime on a lack of resources for prisoners with HIV and other dangerous illnesses, and I will turn to a closer look at the politics of contemporary penal governance and its incongruous relationship to prisoner health and well-being. Later sections of this conclusion draw on recent studies to reflect on the broader impact of mass incarceration on racial inequalities in employment and health care.

Of Race, Punitive Policy, and Catastrophic Prison Health Care

In "Social Construction and Policy Implementation: Inmate Health as a Public Health Issue," Jill and Sean Nicholson-Crotty find significant empirical support for the argument that racialized punitive public policies (such as permanent felon disenfranchisement laws), a lack of African American representation in state legislatures, and stricter welfare provisions result in significantly less state spending on prison health care and services. Moreover, they find "the total number of prisoners negatively correlated with expenditures per inmate, indicating that some states are forced to spend less on inmate care due to their zeal for incarceration."[38] The Nicholson-Crottys also hone in on the impact of state spending for prisoners with HIV/AIDS and tuberculosis (TB). Using data from the Bureau of Justice Statistics (BJS) that includes the number of prisoners infected with HIV in all fifty states, they assess health care expenditures in states with large populations of HIV+ prisoners. Their findings are distressingly all too clear.

> The disturbing finding is that states do not adjust health-care expenditures in response to growing HIV/AIDS and TB rates in the prisons . . . The failure to respond to the increased health care needs of inmates reinforces the conclusion that the negative construction of target groups translates into an under-subscription of benefits, even when the consequences may be life threatening.[39]

To answer the question concerning spending and the comprehensiveness of HIV/AIDS and TB programming in the nation's prisons, the Nicholson-Crottys undertook additional empirical analysis. Using data from the BJS's *National Survey of AIDS in Correctional Facilities,* they analyzed whether comprehensive testing for HIV and TB existed in a particular institution and, looking just at their analysis of HIV/AIDS, the availability of HIV/AIDS education programs recommended by the Centers for Disease Control and the World Health Organization (i.e., concerning safer sex practices and methods for cleaning drug injection equipment). In terms of substantive effects on policy, the Nicholson-Crottys provide convincing evidence.

> These findings provide significant support for the hypothesis that successful implementation of policies designed to mitigate HIV/AIDS and TB requires adequate financial commitment from policymakers . . . Our analysis suggests that one of the *problems* that keeps these sub-objectives [i.e., comprehensive testing and education] from being sufficiently comprehensive is the under-funding that results from the negative construction of the group targeted by these programs.[40]

The Politics of Contemporary Penal Governance

Risk management has become the overriding emphasis for prison managers, an approach that decidedly deemphasizes a focus on prisoner well-being and overemphasizes order maintenance. In the case of Limestone's segregated HIV unit, this has meant an emphasis on security over ensuring humane conditions of confinement. The containment of risk as the dominant managerial strategy has meant less interest in profoundly compromised conditions of confinement and dismal health care delivery and an increased emphasis on minimizing the threat of class action lawsuits. Malcolm Feeley and Van Swearingen contend that the minimizing liability approach is increasingly widespread among penal bureaucrats in the United States more broadly and is "driven by the goal to minimize the threat of litigation, not immediately out of genuine concern over prisoners' conditions of confinement."[41]

At the Interstices of Inequality and Mass Incarceration

Beyond the politics of contemporary penal governance, we must consider the destructiveness of America's accelerated move to address long-standing problems of inequality with incarceration. Rather than confront joblessness and the attendant health care crises in marginalized communities, the most widely embraced approach by policymakers over the last three decades has been to gut health, educational, and employment programs targeted at the poor and focus on the barebones warehousing of such populations. Recent figures documenting growing inequality and the sedimentation of extreme poverty in the United States testify to the continued failure of the nation to confront this economic crisis.[42]

The welfare state has largely been replaced by the penal state. Consider the research of sociologist Bruce Western and colleagues. In an analysis of U.S. Census data between 1980 and 1999 that Western and colleagues adjusted to include prison and jail populations, the employment rate for young black high school dropouts was found to be an astonishingly low 29.9 percent. The authors conclude:

> The great irony of the prison boom is that it comes at a time when policy makers have set out to decrease the role of government in the lives of the disadvantaged. Despite antigovernment rhetoric in policy debates, the government has not regulated the lives of unskilled minority men so intensively since the Depression or wartime . . . The sheer commitment of public resources is comparable in magnitude to social welfare efforts in the 1960s and 1970s. Unlike antipoverty policy, however, the punitive trend in criminal justice policy conceals and deepens economic inequality between blacks and whites.[43]

One must also attend to the "structural violence"—as Paul Farmer terms it—that explains why particular populations are the most vulnerable to the "pattern of neglect and scandal" that continues to characterize many of the nation's jails and prisons today. Importantly, while there has been a pattern—particularly when considering Alabama's jails and prisons—of what Feeley and Swearingen refer to as "half-hearted reform,"[44] very recent transformations in the social and political economies of crime and punishment policy reveal the need to study cases involving the conditions of penal institutions with attention to what Jonathan Simon describes as a country increasingly governed through crime: "Across all kinds of institutional settings, people are seen as acting legitimately when they act to prevent crimes or other troubling behaviors that can be closely analogized to crimes."[45] For marginalized, chronically ill populations, governing through crime has meant what Paul Farmer has called a veritable "war on the poor"; policies that foreclose debate on inadequate health care are replaced with the criminalizing of drug addiction and associated diseases, such as HIV/AIDS and, increasingly, hepatitis C.[46] Known as the "silent epidemic," the number of hepatitis C infections will increase "fourfold" by 2015, according to the National Institutes of Health.[47]

Rather than tackle the real problems of inadequate health care that lead to disproportionately high infant mortality rates, drug and alcohol addiction, and infection rates of deadly diseases, the near wholesale embrace of governing through crime in the majority of American states has trumped governing through health and well-being. Jonathan Simon cogently explains: "The story is less one of extending state power through crime than it is one in which the importance the state has assigned to crime nudges out other kinds of opportunities that a different hierarchy of public problems might produce—e.g., a government obsessed with governing by educating would produce all kinds of incentives to define various people as efficient or deficient in education."[48] The state's dedication of exorbitant financial resources to being tough on crime through mass incarceration policies all but forecloses the opportunity of the state to invest in better education and employment opportunities and health care in poor, often racially aggrieved communities.

From Declining Penal Welfare to Declining Health Welfare

In actuality, mass incarceration and the erosion of public accountability have led many U.S. states to reembrace the inhumane, captive institutions that were aggressively attacked by reformers in the 1970s. Indeed, the current state of affairs is more akin to the often brutal institutions that were characteristic of a time preceding the progressive reforms at the turn of the twentieth century. In short, the last three decades have increasingly been characterized by a nationalistic fear of crime and an ideology of control characterized by a focus on containing threatening populations—what sociologist David Garland calls the rise of a "crime complex"[49]—as opposed to a more localized view of crime as a community problem that could only be addressed by focusing on the rehabilitation of individuals so they could reenter their communities as law-abiding citizens.

Obviously, this view—what Garland calls "penal welfarism"—is more than a little naive, as David Rothman illustrates in his compelling study of the failed attempts of progressive reformers to employ an idealistic, conscience-driven approach to grappling with crime and other social problems.[50] To build on Rothman's famous phrase "conscience and convenience," progressive consciousness of rehabilitation and care invariably gave way to impersonal, often corrosively politicized bureaucratic convenience. If the Progressive Era taught anything about penal institutions, it was, as Rothman concludes, the failure to create penal institutions that were humane. Yet the lessons of Progressive Era incarceration—namely, the need to put fewer people in captive institutions—has obviously fallen on deaf ears in the last three decades.

Especially since the early 1980s, a declining concern with penal welfarism has also meant a declining concern with "health welfarism." In his first months in office, President Reagan made the largest tax cuts and investments in corporate welfare in the nation's history, while simultaneously gutting vital programs for the poor and racially aggrieved, "especially," as W. Michael Byrd and Linda Clayton note in *An American Health Dilemma*, "expenditures for their health care."[51] Byrd and Clayton explain that subsequent inflation as the result of huge increases on defense spending and the attendant mountain of federal debt "adversely impacted the health of Blacks and the poor by decreasing city tax bases, revenues, and funding sources for the nation's already fragile public health infrastructure composed of public and charity clinics and city and county hospitals."[52]

The veritable evisceration of health care for the poor that continued throughout the eighties and into the present—despite the nation's dwindling numbers of often cash-strapped nonprofit temporary care facilities—emboldened the rise of what Vicente Navarro and colleagues famously foresaw in 1967 as the "medical industrial complex."[53] As documented by Byrd and Clayton, this system is driven by a for-profit, "bottom-line" mentality that has had profound implications for governing the health of marginalized populations more broadly: "For African Americans, Hispanic/Latino Americans, and other disadvantaged ethnic groups, the working class (almost 75 percent of the population), those with chronic illnesses who do not have adequate public or third-party coverage, and the poor in the health system, such a transformed medical industrial complex represents a threatening and potentially hostile new health care environment."[54] Byrd and Clayton also provide comprehensive documentation of the current black/white disparity in life expectancy, a disparity that increased dramatically in the twelve years of the Reagan and George H. W. Bush presidencies. This prison of concentrated poverty and the defunding of health care for the poor in the United States has meant (to name but a very few racial disparities in health) that blacks in the United States today remain 3.3 times more likely than whites to die of AIDS, 2.3 times more likely to die of diabetes mellitus, and 1.3 times as likely to die from chronic liver disease and cirrhosis.[55]

Mass incarceration is a portal into what Susan Sered and Rushika Fernandopulle term America's health care "death spiral." How a catchy phrase like "prison of concentrated poverty" (which I use in the preceding paragraph) is realized in the lives of chronically ill Americans who lack health insurance is documented in Sered and Fernandopulle's *Uninsured in America: Life and Death in the Land of Opportunity.* Drawing on extensive interviews with 120 uninsured Americans from Texas, Mississippi, Idaho, Illinois, and Massachusetts, Sered and Fernandopulle present a chilling portrait of the death spiral. Beyond insurance lingo and catchy metaphors, Sered and Fernandopulle demonstrate a deadly, downward trajectory among the uninsured that "can easily lead to health concerns going untreated, a situation that can exacerbate employment problems by making the individual less able to work." Sered and Fenandopulle continue: "Alternatively, the downward spiral can begin with health problems that lead to employment problems making it less likely that one will have health insurance and thus reducing the chances of solving the original health issues."[56]

Sered and Fernandopulle document pathways for entering into the health care death spiral. One such portal is prison. But beyond typical allusions to high prisoner death rates, their analysis of prison as linked to failed health care policy in the United States is important for a deeper understanding of the connection between criminal justice and inequality. Sered and Fernandopulle articulate how felony status for a chronically ill person may mean lack of employment and, in turn, lack of treatment.

In a pattern typical of the death spiral, we fill our prisons largely with people who have committed petty (mostly drug-related) crimes. We re-classify many of these crimes as felonies, which means that, once re-leased, the former prisoners cannot find reasonable employment. Thus, they lack access to health care, which means that they get sick(er), which means that they need to find ways legal or not to obtain life's necessities, including medication. And they end up back in jail, sicker than before.[57]

Investments in "Us and Them"

If the Limestone case has taught anything at all, it is that recent con-ventional wisdom about prisoners, which drove more than three decades of mass incarceration policies, has been corrosive to Ameri-can democracy. The ideology of "us and them" that drove the recent punishment wave not only creates a phony separation between chron-ically ill prisoners and poor, often racially aggrieved populations living outside prison walls. It also drives a wedge between "them" and "us"— that is, the majority of Americans who are presently not kept in cap-tive institutions and who live far away from the prisons of educational inequality, joblessness, and lack of health insurance.

The story of more than thirty years of mass imprisonment in the contemporary United States is fraught with injustice, needless suffer-ing, and preventable deaths. As has been well documented, it is no co-incidence that such a state of affairs has expanded dramatically with a continued failure on the part of policymakers to address the health care crisis in marginalized communities.[58] The story told throughout this book forces one to confront a not particularly pleasant truth: we live in a world today where it is acceptable that enormous numbers of human beings are warehoused far away from public view and allowed to needlessly suffer and die.

Beyond the obvious problems associated with captive institutions, these policies have meant a deepening loss of public accountability and broader investments in a captive society. The recent scandalous treatment of severely injured Iraq War veterans at the Walter Reed Army Medical Center is a glaring example of this increasing trend. Slashing public funds for wounded veterans is the result of a profound loss of public accountability, accelerated particularly over the past three decades. In a word, cost cutting has trumped genuine care for those powerless to challenge the conditions of their surroundings. Despite all we have known about catastrophes associated with captive bureaucracies—inside nursing homes, VA hospitals, and youth reform schools—we have largely chosen to ignore these institutions until the next disaster strikes, until the next whistle-blower dares to come forward.

Beyond high-profile scandals are the entrenched conditions of American apartheid that continue to loom large in this era of deregulated civil rights. Despite the continued legacies of denial and blame that nourish what might best be called the "clearest manifestations" of the captive society today—staggering numbers of isolated Americans still without basic health care or access to quality education and gainful employment—the subject only enters into the public discourse in the wake of such monumental catastrophes as Hurricane Katrina's decimation of the poorest communities in Louisiana and the Mississippi Gulf Coast.[59] Even in the wake of widespread public attention, windows into the enduring captive landscape of American inequality were quickly shut, and attention turned to the "blame game" rhetoric of *Fox News* pundit Bill O'Reilly[60] and the policy blunders of political elites. Most consequentially, the focus of public policy in the wake of Hurricane Katrina quickly became aggressive cost cutting, doing disaster relief on the cheap, and corporate profiteering run amok. The Bush administration's central strategy for dealing with the aftermath of the Gulf Coast crises has been to offer no-bid contracts to for-profit service providers—contracts that, according to a recent report from the U.S. Government Accountability Office, have resulted in at least two billion dollars in fraud.[61]

The Continued Struggle for HIV+ Prisoners

The current system severely damages the people it imprisons and the communities most affected by it. We promote alternatives to policing and prisons and challenge the prison industrial com-

plex in all its forms. We fulfill our mission by: Providing legal services and supporting prisoner
organizing efforts that promote health and justice; Working with prisoners, their families and
community members on political education and mobilization campaigns; Building coalitions
to create safety for women and individual accountability without relying on the punishment
system; Training the next generation of activists and lawyers committed to working for social
justice.

—JUSTICE NOW

A hopeful sign for HIV+ prisoners is the remarkable work of non-profit organizations working inside and outside the nation's jails and prisons today (see appendix C for a list of prisoner activist organizations in the United States). One of the most effective organizations in the United States is Justice Now, a nonprofit activist-centered prisoner rights organization (formerly the Women's Positive Legal Action Network) based in Oakland, California. Justice Now represents an important development in post-PLRA prisoner rights advocacy, one that reemphasizes the objectives of early prisoner activists. Specifically, Justice Now takes a broad approach to confronting HIV/AIDS behind bars by putting prisoners at the center of the organization's mission.

Cofounder Cynthia Chandler explains Justice Now's approach as follows:

> We are really committed to this idea that prisoners are the ones who guide the strategy work. So having those kinds of close, but always professional, relationships to people is necessary to gain their trust, to get them to feel like they can actually be part of the process. We are really committed to involving prisoners in this broader campaign work and abolitionist work that we are doing. We want prisoners to direct it and be very much a part of it . . . I feel that one of the reasons that the actual legal work that we do is so important is that it actually doesn't contradict, but actually goes well with, that broader systemic work.[62]

Chandler takes a realistic view of Justice Now's broader commitment to prison abolition.

> On one level, you just can't go and ask a prisoner a crazy question like, "What would it take to build a world without prisons?"—especially if

their arm is rotting off; or if they have just lost their children and they don't know what to do to appeal it, or they may never be able to see their kid again; or they are losing their eyesight because their retina is detaching, and they only have twenty-four hours left to get their vision back. Prisoners don't have the intellectual luxury to theorize that kind of stuff; they don't have the luxury if they are experiencing enormous suffering. So I feel like it is essential to do work to address people's day-to-day concerns and their real suffering, in order to give people the ability to do that other kind of work. And so that is important.

Chandler views prisoner involvement as a way to both empower individual prisoners and build a broader community of activists.

Also I think that many of the prisoners that we work with have come to us already saying that they want to be activists, or they are already activists within the prisons. But other people come to us with these dire needs, and then it's this process of us getting them information about their health so that they can direct the work that we do for them. It is then that they get really empowered and start wanting to help other people. We frequently see the birth of new activists actively involved in their own legal assistance. So it is really part of a whole leadership development process as well, finding ways to combine doing the direct service work with avenues for people involved in broader social change.

EPILOGUE

As *Birmingham News* reporter Carla Crowder sat down with former Limestone prisoner Wilson Rogers[1] in a park across the street from Birmingham's famous rib joint Dreamland, an Alabama culinary treasure located among the bustling bars and coffee shops in the trendy Five Points South, she couldn't help but be surprised at how upbeat and healthy Rogers looked: "He was very poised and spoke with ease about the deaths." Dressed in neatly pressed shorts, a designer golf shirt, and gold chains, Rogers was a lively, articulate speaker, living in the Fellowship House, a large sixty-day coed transitional living center for the recently paroled, those in need of drug treatment, or both. Located in the Southside of Birmingham, in an eclectic neighborhood comprised of once-grand old Victorians and cheap college student apartments, as well as churches, social services agencies, and other group homes, the Fellowship House was founded in 1973, a period of strong federal support for public health.

Hundreds of such facilities closed as a result of defunding beginning in the Reagan years, but Fellowship House was able to independently incorporate as a nonprofit and has provided a host of outpatient services and residential programs for more than three decades.[2] For Rogers, such vital services have meant dramatic improvements in his health.

My health is doing real well. My T cell count is up. I'm not stressing. And, again, I try to eat better now that I'm out, a lot of salads and fruits; and I drink a lot of water. So it's better than it has been. I've never been sick, and that's only by the grace of God. But I'm doing the things that I need to do now . . . For medicines, I only take a combination of three pills, and that's something that I just recently started, and it's working real well.

But Rogers's sixty days at the Fellowship House would be over soon, and he planned to move in with his sister in Montgomery. "It's always a challenge," he said, "but I'm so close with my family, I'm hopeful for the future."

Michael Ramsey, another former Limestone prisoner, now lives in a tidy, white, frame house in a working-class and low-income neighborhood called East Lake. The Aletheia House, a rehab and transitional living program in which he is enrolled, owns the home. It is sparsely furnished with secondhand furniture. But Ramsey's comfortable there, as it's obviously a step up from most places he has lived. He lives on a side street, within walking distance of a convenience store and fast-food restaurants.

For her interview with Ramsey, Crowder sat outside on a small front porch, so Ramsey could smoke. He shook a cigarette out immediately but mostly just used it to gesture. Ramsey's most distinguishing feature are his large, sad, puppy dog eyes. Crowder observed:

> He uses them to ask for help. While talking with him, he needed help understanding the documents associated with a recent accident in which he was struck by a car in a mall parking lot. He is average height, slightly paunchy. Dressed in an old T-shirt and sweat pants, Ramsey, because of his poverty and health problems, almost seems trapped in that little house. But he has friends from the Aletheia program who come by to visit, so he seems strangely content, considering the simplicity of his life.

Crowder's interview with Ramsey revealed that despite a bit of a rocky road since his parole, Ramsey's faith enables him to stay committed to living.

RAMSEY: I'm going to live until God is ready for me. But I ain't going to die. I'm going to pray, and with the grace of God, I'm not going to die with this virus. I'm going to try to take care of myself and try to live as long as I can. So if I die, it's cuz God's ready for me. Whether a heart attack, car wreck, or something like that, he'll be ready. But it ain't going to be cuz of this virus. I refuse to let the virus kill me. I take care of myself, and as long as I don't mess with them drugs, the virus won't kill me. I don't know what stage I'm in now. But whatever stage I'm in, I'm fighting.

CROWDER: What brings happiness to you now? I mean, what do you do for fun, to make life worth living?

RAMSEY: Well, with the grace of God, I don't use drugs no more, so I just like TV and listening to music. I got a friend; he's still in prison. He should be getting out this year or definitely next year. And I'm just sitting back, just chillin' out, waiting on him. I just live as days go by. And I'm alright without friends. You know, if I meet a friend or we go out to the movies or something, that is alright, too. But if I don't meet anyone, I still like being by myself like this everyday. I'm comfortable with that. And I've been in the streets before. I know how it is: not good.

The stories of Rogers and Ramsey and of the forty-three HIV+ prisoners at Limestone and hundreds of others who have perished behind bars are tales that most Americans are unlikely to have heard before. Indeed, most Americans might say they "don't need to know," as "that could never happen" to them. According to a recent report from the Bureau of Justice Statistics, between 2001 and 2004, a staggering 870 prisoners died of AIDS-related complications inside U.S. prisons.[3] It is likely that hundreds more incarcerated with the virus in the nation's jails have died as well. Their identities are shrouded in the secrecy of increasingly catastrophic penal bureaucracies. These men and women are people that most of us will likely never know. Their deaths are recorded, if at all, in sloppily written, incomplete penal death records.

"The Futility of Severe Punishment and Cruel Treatment"

It is the overriding hope of this book that more Americans, perhaps even policymakers, will want—indeed, demand—to know how those in U.S. captive institutions are treated. In order to prevent future catastrophes, more people must know. In the case of disabled veterans and prisoners respectively, ignorance will only lead to more tragedies like those at Walter Reed and Limestone. Sadly, it is likely already far too late. Perhaps for disabled veterans, recent congressional investigations will result in less constraint and better care for those currently trapped in the nation's grossly substandard VA medical bureaucracies.[4]

In the case of penal institutions, we confront another challenge: humanizing those who have broken the law and replacing hysteria and rage with justice and pragmatism. This will doubtlessly entail dramatic decreases in the use of incarceration as a tool for addressing long-standing inequalities and injustices in the nation and the wherewithal to fight for employment and education opportunities and humane health care for all, regardless of prison status, race, class, gender, age, disability, or sexuality. By doing so, the hope is that we will increase the transparency of the captive, often catastrophic institutions that needlessly hide away so many of our sick and dying citizens. The powerful effect of transparency vis-à-vis activism and the media has been demonstrated by the compelling story of Jerome Miller, former head of the Massachusetts juvenile justice system, who exhibited bold internal leadership in his successful closing of grossly inhumane juvenile reform schools in Massachusetts. The hope is that more inhumane captive institutions will eventually shut their doors.

None of the goals I have advocated are likely to be met in the immediate future. The challenges are large and complex. This is especially the case in a society whose leaders have turned their backs on deepening inequalities in health, education, and employment, at the same time that they have aggressively embraced grossly inhumane mass imprisonment policies. In the classic *Punishment and Social Structure,* sociologists George Rusche and Otto Kircheimer presciently observed some seventy years ago:

> The futility of severe punishment and cruel treatment may be proven a thousand times, but so long as society is unable to solve its social problems, repression, the easy way out, will always be accepted. It provides the *illusion of security* by covering the symptoms of social disease with a system of legal and moral value judgments.[5]

APPENDIX A

A Fuller Account of Methods

In the fall of 2002, I set out to learn more about the effects of the Prisoner Litigation Reform Act of 1995 (PLRA) on prisoner rights advocacy. A colleague from a nearby law school in Philadelphia directed to me to the Southern Center for Human Rights (SCHR). My initial interview was done over the phone with Tamara Serwer, an SCHR attorney who had recent experience with a post-PLRA case involving HIV+ prisoners at Georgia's Fulton County Jail. The questioning was conceived around Catherine Kohler Riessman's qualitative methods volume on narrative analysis. Specifically, I was interested in collecting stories about post-PLRA prisoner rights advocacy, so my questions were worded very broadly (e.g., "Tell me about your experiences working on prisoner rights cases since the passage of the PLRA").

I did not intend to focus on HIV+ prisoners specifically. But after the first interview with Serwer, I became increasingly interested in this especially vulnerable population. From there, I decided to use a snowball sampling technique, as Serwer informed me that, given dwindling resources and recent closings of many prisoner rights organizations, it was important to get in touch with key actors presently involved in the issue. I also became very interested in the prisoner's perspective, as Serwer spoke very passionately about the crucial role prisoners played in all phases of litigation. Knowing that it would be next to impossible to get approval from my institution's institutional review board (or, for that matter, the consent of various jail and prison officials) to interview HIV+ prisoners on-site, I knew it would be very important for me to find informant(s) who worked closely with the prisoners, particularly in Alabama.

Until Serwer had mentioned it to me, I knew absolutely nothing about the Limestone case. She mentioned that she had recently turned her attention to it, and she gave me a brief overview of the facts, but she informed me that new SCHR attorney Joshua Lipman had taken the lead on the case and that it was crucial for me to interview him. I would eventually interview Lipman several weeks later, but at the time, I still had no intention of doing a case study. Serwer directed me to also speak with sociologist and longtime prisoner rights activist Rachel Maddow.

My interview with Rachel was a huge breakthrough. Not only did she provide me with a list of activists and lawyers currently involved in issues concerning HIV+ prisoners, but she gave me invaluable insights into the contours of the struggle, especially from the perspective of social movements. Maddow had just finished her sociology dissertation at Oxford on activist work for HIV+ prisoners in the United Kingdom and the United States, and she graciously sent the entire document to me only weeks later. Reading Maddow's dissertation made it clear that I needed to ask more questions about the role of current prisoners and ex-prisoners in advocacy and litigation. Moreover, she told me about her current position with the ACLU and about the "No Lost Causes" conference.

After publishing an article and a chapter on the more than twenty interviews I had conducted with advocates who had worked on post-PLRA cases involving HIV+ prisoners from around the United States (some of this data is used in chapter 4), I was still stuck with a central question: how could a monumental catastrophe such as Limestone have taken place? I knew that the PLRA had some role in blocking Lipman and his colleagues, but as a sociologist interested in organizations, I also became convinced that there were broader structural factors that I needed to get a better handle on. First, I turned to the literature on mass incarceration policies, prison health, and the state of health care for the poor, as I knew there were important connections to be made. This literature was very helpful but often cast southern prisons too simplistically, in what I perceived as overly negative terms. I knew from my interviews with respondents from the Northeast that there were a lot of serious problems in penal institutions from that region of the country, so this literature was very useful for capturing the broad picture but more limited in terms of exploring the issues from below.

I then decided to take a trip to Atlanta to meet with members of SCHR in person. Those two days were extremely fruitful and convinced me that the Limestone case needed to be told. SCHR provided me with public documents and local Alabama news accounts of the case, which left me with the impression that the case was about overtly deviant practices on the part of for-profit medical providers. The literature I had read seemed to confirm that assumption over and over again. But I still felt too distanced from Alabama to really know what had happened there.

One of the most interesting articles that I obtained from SCHR was by *Birmingham News* journalist Carla Crowder. Her piece stood out to me because it was a broad political critique of Limestone in the context of Alabama politics but was written by someone who obviously had intimate knowledge of the case from a local perspective. After subsequent e-mail exchanges with Carla, she agreed to share with me all she knew about the case and various leads to follow. For example, I knew nothing about Alabama's regressive tax system, public health problems around HIV/AIDS, or the details surrounding the hiring of Naphcare.

Only after several long phone conversations with Carla did I begin to see the emergence of a more complex picture of the Limestone case. Moreover, and perhaps most important, I had contacted Carla when she was still very much engaged in the Limestone case, and she graciously offered to let me read early versions of her own work as well as interviews she would subsequently conduct with ex-prisoners. I could not have written this book without Carla's invaluable assistance and also her willingness to read early drafts of the manuscript.

By early 2005, I had completed what I thought was a nearly finished manuscript. But I wanted to read other sociological case studies that were recently published, to get a better sense conceptually of what these scholars had accomplished. To some extent, I felt that my manuscript was a bit too one-dimensional. I thought that reading other works might either dispel that feeling or provide me with new analytical directions worth pursuing.

I read the work of Diane Vaughan, Jerome Miller, Michel Richard, and Eric Klinenberg, as well as, most recently, Susanne Monahan and Beth Quin's case study of the Abu Ghraib prison catastrophe. These works influenced me to thoroughly revisit my own project. They really pushed me to reconsider the current "deviant individuals" narrative I had crafted and especially to probe deeper into Dr. Tabet's massive report. The closer I analyzed that document and learned about the subsequent internal issues surrounding individual staff members, Alabama politics, and the fact that some states (e.g., Rhode Island) had, for all intents and purposes, quality prison health care for HIV+ prisoners, the more I realized that Limestone was far more a story of deviant institutional practices than one of "bad apples" and "evil leaders."

I developed a coding scheme to analyze Dr. Tabet's report for patterns in institutional practices in Limestone's Health Care Unit (see the results in chapter 6). I then began to do systematic analysis of media reports on other state penal institutions, in order to learn if the kinds of problems that were occurring were indicative of my theory of catastrophic institutional failure. After reviewing hundreds of articles—the majority of which were "prison horror stories"—I found several reports of institutional failures that went well beyond the story of "deviant individuals" that I was initially wed to. While I can no way claim that the analysis in appendix B is exhaustive, it at least confirmed for me that there was a bigger picture that was presently missing from my current manuscript.

Drawing on Dianne Vaughan's insight—in appendix C of her magisterial and awe-inspiring book *The Challenger Launch Decision*—to explore institutional overlap in the processes between other institutions, I turned to other studies for insights. I was familiar with Goffman's classic work in *Asylums*, but I felt as though it was a bit too detached from the subjects under scrutiny. While I agreed with Goffman's overall conception of the total institution, I also agreed with Michel Richard's claim, in his insightful essay "Goffman Revisited: Relatives vs. Administrators in Nursing Homes," that Goffman had not paid close enough attention to contingencies involving personnel (e.g., I knew that Dr. Chijide was far more complex than a static agent of control) and that prisoners were far less passive "victims" than Goffman seemingly believed (see chapter 6, "Creating Alternative Spaces of Care"). Studies by Susanne Monahan and Beth Quin (on Abu Ghraib prison), Michel Richard (on nursing homes), Jerome Miller (on juvenile reform schools), and Jonathan Shay (on traumatized Vietnam veterans) provided far thicker descriptions than Goffman's work and thus proved extremely helpful to me in further crystallizing the book's central theme of "catastrophic penal institutions."

APPENDIX B

The Institutional Lives of Catastrophic Jails and Prisons in the United States, 1990–2007

The information in this appendix comes from systematic searches of the Nexus news database between 1990 and 2007. The analysis was designed to learn more about recent institutional failures in prisons and jails from around the United States. While many of the articles I discovered did not provide the kind of sociological insight I was looking for—that is, many focused on isolated incidents—several excellent in-depth investigative reports provided me with thicker descriptions of institutional problems associated with penal health bureaucracies in the contemporary United States. Obviously, I cannot claim that these "snapshots" of institutional failure prove my contention that there has been an influx in the last thirty years in the number of penal institutions that can justifiably be called "catastrophic." But I do believe that the reports at least suggest this observation.

SOUTHWEST

Arizona

There are numerous reports of institutional failures in Arizona's penal institutions, including the normalization of deviant practices at Sheriff Joseph Arpaio's notorious tent city jails. Between 1993 and 1996, eleven prisoners died in custody in Maricopa County's infamous Ward 41. According to a report in the *Phoenix New Times,* one prisoner, Jose Rodriquez died of untreated heroin detoxification, "curled up on a mattress on a concrete floor, his head resting in his own vomit."[1] The report stated that despite being surrounded by hundreds of people, including trained medical personnel, Rodriquez was ignored and accused of faking his ailment.

Texas

Although prison health care in Texas has been touted as "a model for the nation," a 2001 investigative report conducted by journalists from the *Houston Press* documented the negative findings of recent state audits.[2] The audits revealed medical personnel discouraging prisoners from obtaining medication, doctors at local prison units routinely ignoring the assessments of health specialists, a rise in infectious diseases (e.g., hepatitis, tuberculosis, and drug-resistant staph), and serious lapses in treatment for HIV and AIDS. Moreover, according to the report, an audit of prisoner deaths in the state in 1998 concluded that twenty of the inmates "received poor or very poor care" and that the deaths of sixteen of those twenty inmates were either "preventable" or "possibly preventable."[3]

SOUTH

Arkansas

An audit of Correctional Medical Services, conducted by the U.S. Justice Department between July and September of 2002, found that Arkansas prisoners did not receive proper referral or follow-up services and that medical services were grossly understaffed, lacked supervision, and failed to consistently implement medical policies and protocols.[4]

Florida

In January 2007, the Pinellas County Jail, a Florida facility built to hold twenty-four hundred men and women, held a population of thirty-eight hundred prisoners. One investigator reported:

> Hundreds must sleep in portable beds on the floor, often next to toilets or beneath sinks. The infirmary, designed for 44, usually has 70 to 80 inmates a day. Those with nonessential medical needs often wait months to be treated. When a contagious disease such as chickenpox breaks out, the staff quarantines the entire cellblock and lets the disease run its course.[5]

WEST

Colorado

As of 2002, three thousand Colorado prisoners had tested positive for hepatitis C, but only thirty-four received any drug therapy. A report in the *Denver Westword* profiled one prisoner, Terry Akers, who was denied treatment.

> Last spring his stomach became grossly distended, as if he were carrying a beach ball under his shirt. At first the doctors suspected a bacterial infection, but it was ascites, an accumulation of fluid that is one of the common symptoms of cirrhosis. The veins in his esophagus also became painfully swollen. The DOC's internal medicine specialist said he'd seen worse. After dinner a couple of months ago, Akers began to vomit blood.

A physician's assistant responded to his distress call, looked in his toilet and decided, yep, that was a lot of blood . . . Terry Akers's esophogeal varices had ruptured in five places, requiring surgery.[6]

Utah

An investigation of the Point of the Mountain prison in Utah revealed gross neglect of prisoners with mental illness. According to a 1997 report in the *Salt Lake Tribune*, prison staff routinely used a device known as "the chair" as a means for brutally controlling mentally ill prisoners.

Many are stripped naked and hooked to a catheter while subjected to sit-down confinement. On March 20, 1997, mentally ill inmate Michael Valent spent about 16 of the last 18 hours of his life strapped to the chair. He died of a pulmonary embolism brought on by the restraint.[7]

NORTHEAST

New York

In 2005, troubling reports surfaced surrounding the deaths of twenty-four prisoners in ten New York City Jails under care of Prison Health Services. A New York State commission attributed the deaths to poorly kept medical records, poorly dispensed medications, inadequate staff, and erratic care.[8]

New Hampshire

According to one news report, an audit conducted of prison health care in New Hampshire in 2003 by the Legislative Budget Assistant's Office described the system as having an "ineffective organizational structure, incompetent management and insufficient oversight of the quality of care."[9]

MIDWEST

Nebraska

A 2000 report on Nebraska's prison medical care system by state ombudsman Marshall Lux discovered numerous systemic problems, including "poor treatment of cardiac patients, faulty administration of pain medication, lack of staff training, and medical decisions based on fiscal concerns."[10]

Iowa

A 1999 investigative report and interview with Iowa ombudsman William P. Angrick revealed that there were nine doctors assigned to care for the state's seventy-one hundred prisoners. The investigator reported that mentally ill prisoners at Fort Madison prison were segregated in the chaotic Cellblock

220, a place where prisoners were given little treatment, often abandoned, and subjected to "maddening waves of noise."[11]

New Jersey

A 2004 audit of New Jersey's prison mental health services revealed numerous institutional failures. A national expert in prison mental health, Dennis Koson, described the state of treatment for mentally ill prisoners in New Jersey as "the worst I have seen in my 15 years of inspecting correctional systems nationwide."[12]

Maryland

As of March 2007, an audit of Maryland's penal system conducted by the Office of Legislative Audits concluded that providers of medical care, dental care, and mental health care were grossly understaffed and had many "problems with medical screenings, chronic care checkups, medication dispensation and timely treatment based on inmate needs."[13]

APPENDIX C

Prisoner Activism and Advocacy Organizations in North America

Critical Resistance
National Office
1904 Franklin Street, Suite 504
Oakland, CA 94612
http://criticalresistance.org

Justice Now
1322 Webster Street, Suite 210
Oakland, CA 94612
http://www.justicenow.org

Stop Prison Rape
3325 Wilshire Boulevard, Suite 340
Los Angeles, CA 90010
http://spr.org

National Prison Hospice Association
PO Box 55
Lafayette, CO
http://www.npha.org

Delaware Center for Justice
501 Shipley Street
Wilmington, DE 19801
http://dcjustice.org

Alliance for Inmates with AIDS
80 Fifth Avenue, Suite 1501
New York, NY 10011

Positive People on Parole (POP)
The Speilman Center
415 West Fifty-first Street
New York, NY 10019

Prisoners with AIDS Support Action Network (PASAN)
517 College Street, Suite 237
Toronto, ON M6G 4A2

Hepatitis C Awareness Project
Phyllis Beck, Director
PO Box 41803
Eugene, OR 97404
http://hcvinprison.org

PRISONER LEGAL SERVICES

Alabama Prison Project
215 Clayton Street
Montgomery, AL 36104

Equal Justice Initiative
122 Commerce Street
Montgomery, AL 36104
http://eji.org

Legal Services for Prisoners with Children
1540 Market Street, Suite 490
San Francisco, CA 94102
http://www.prisonerswithchildren.org

American Civil Liberties Union
National Prison Project
1875 Connecticut Avenue NW, Suite 410
Washington, DC 20009
http://www.aclu.org/prison/index.html

Southern Center for Human Rights
83 Poplar Street NW
Atlanta, GA 30303
http://www.schr.org

Massachusetts Correctional Legal Services (MCLS)
8 Winter Street
Boston, MA 02108
http://www.mcls.net

Prisoners' Legal Services of New York (PLS)
105 Chambers Street, Fifth Floor
New York, NY 10007
http://www.plsny.org

North Carolina Prisoner Legal Services, Inc.
PO Box 25397
Raleigh, NC 27611
http://www.ncpls.org

AIDS Law Project of Pennsylvania
1211 Chestnut Street, Suite 1200
Philadelphia, PA 19107

RESEARCH AND HEALTH ADVOCACY

HIV in Prisons Program
Yale AIDS Program
135 College Street, Suite 323
New Haven, CT 06510
http://yalemedicine.yale.edu/ym_su98/cover/cov_prison08.html

The Sentencing Project
514 Tenth Street NW, Suite 1000
Washington, DC 20004
http://www.sentencingproject.org

National Commission on Correctional Health Care
1145 W. Diversey Parkway
Chicago, IL 60614
http://www.ncchc.org

Abt Associates Inc.
55 Wheeler Street
Cambridge, MA 02138
http://www.abtassociates.com

NOTES

INTRODUCTION

1. Throughout this book, I use both the terms *jail* and *prison* when discussing broader problems surrounding health care behind bars. It is important to distinguish the two institutions, as jails not only are penal institutions but are also used as lawful houses of detention. Moreover, jails are run at the local levels of county or city government. Because local governments are especially likely to lack adequate resources to deal with the problems of overcrowding and to provide adequate care to chronically ill prisoners, this distinction is important when one realizes just how catastrophic health care conditions have become in so many U.S. jails.

2. Whitman 1990, 20–26.

3. Ibid., 21.

4. To ensure anonymity, Whitman changed last names of all prisoners and guards profiled in the article.

5. Whitman 1990, 20.

6. Ibid., 22.

7. Ibid., 26.

8. The 1998 feature, by correspondent Aram Roston, is available online at http://www.cnn.com/US/9812/22/hiv.prisoners/index.html.

9. Acton 2000.

10. Ibid., A5.

11. See Sloop 1996 for an exhaustive analysis of fifty years of popular discourse on prisoners in the United States. Sloop's analysis reveals profoundly distorted, often racialized popular constructions of prisoners, especially in recent popular press accounts.

12. This lack in detailed media coverage may very well exist principally because of high access barriers set by prison authorities. Moreover, cutbacks in news coverage have resulted in few newspapers that are able to have reporters regularly assigned to cover the prison beat. For a detailed report of these developments, see "Silencing the Oppressed: No Freedom of Speech for Those behind the Walls," available online from Prison Legal News, at http://www. prisonlegalnews.org/2505_displayArticle.aspx.

13. Zimring and Hawkins (1991) were among the first to systematically analyze the increases in the U.S. prison population. For more recent studies that shed important light on the rise of mass incarceration policies at the national level, see Western 2006; Garland 2001b; Gottschalk 2006; Beckett 1997. Regarding state-level analyses, Vanessa Barker (2006) has conducted an important analysis that demonstrates how variations in state-level governance shed light on why some states incarcerate more aggressively than others.

14. Curiously, there have not been very many ethnographic studies of prisons in America. In a recent special issue of the journal *Ethnography,* sociologist Loïc Wacquant (2002, 385) observes, "Observational studies depicting the everyday world of inmates all but vanished just as the U.S. was settling into mass incarceration and other advanced countries were gingerly clearing their own road towards the penal state." The same issue presents several contemporary ethnographies of the prison in the United States (Jacobson-Hardy 2002; Comfort 2002; Gowan 2002: see also Rhodes 2004), Brazil (Goifman 2002), and France (Marchetti 2002). For a contemporary ethnographic study of women prisoners in the United States, see McCorkel forthcoming. For an engaging ethnography of parole officers in California, see Lynch 1998.

15. I was not able to do observation within the prison. Instead, I rely on extensive interviews with attorneys and activists, analysis of extensive archival materials, and one particularly important informant, who became my principle collaborator on this work. For a more detailed discussion of methods, see appendix A.

16. Klinenberg 2003, 23.

CHAPTER 1

1. Rusche and Kirchheimer [1939] 1968; Clemmer 1940.

2. Sykes [1958] 1974, 8. Other pathbreaking ethnographic and historical studies of penal institutions include Irwin [1970] 1987; Rothman [1971] 2002b; Rothman [1980] 2002a; S. Cohen 1985.

3. J. Jacobs 1977, 203.

4. Ibid., 136. For studies demonstrating the power of law to mobilize rights in the workplace, see McCann 1994.

5. Throughout this book, my use of the term *total institution* draws on the conception of Rose, Glazer, and Glazer (1977, 375), which emphasizes controlled environments. For an essay on the career of the "total institution" as a sociological concept, see C. A. McEwen 1980.

6. Goffman 1961.

7. For an excellent volume detailing the myriad intended and unintended consequences of mass incarceration policies, see Mauer and Chesney-Lind

2002. On the broader social and political dimensions of these policies, see Garland 2001b.

8. New York State Special Commission on Attica 1972, 65–66.

9. Sered and Fernandopulle 2005, 213.

10. Starr 1982, 420–49.

11. Byrd and Clayton 2002, 496.

12. McDonald 1999, 457.

13. In an influential essay, Burawoy (1998, 5) explains, "The extended case method applies reflexive science to ethnography in order to extract the general from the unique, to move the 'micro' to the 'macro,' and to connect the present to the past in anticipation of the future, all by building on preexisting theory." I aspire to the aims of Burawoy, but as a nontraditional ethnographer interested in events that have already occurred, my approach to the extended case study is more analogous to historical ethnography, as I was not a participant observer at the time of the deaths at Limestone prison.

14. For compelling analyses of the early years of the AIDS epidemic, exploring both ideological and bureaucratic dimensions of the crisis, see Perrow and Guillén 1990; Musheno, Gregware, and Drass 1991.

15. For analyses of AIDS narratives and how they were visually represented in the mainstream press, see Treichler 1999; Albertini 2004; Gilman 1987.

16. Many commentators have linked the chaos to the widespread war on drugs. A leading scholar of prison law, Ralf Jurgens (1994, 786), observes:

In the United States, the "war on drugs" has been ongoing inside and outside prisons for many years and has had a profound impact on prisons generally and on the approach to HIV/AIDS and drug use in prisons specifically. The major outcome of the war on drugs has not been a reduction in use, trafficking, and drug-related crime, but a dramatic increase in incarceration rates.

17. Liptak 2003; Crowder 2002, 2003, 2004, 2005, 2006.

18. Crowder 2006.

19. Reporters from the *Milwaukee Journal Sentinel* conducted an eight-month investigation of every prisoner death in Wisconsin between 1994 and 2000. See Zahn and McBride 2000.

20. Dr. Tabet conducted two separate evaluations. The first, conducted on August 23, 2003, documented the physical examinations of nineteen prisoners who were living at Dorm 16 at the time of Dr. Tabet's visit and thirty-eight mortality reviews of HIV+ prisoners who had died between 1999 and 2003. The second evaluation, conducted on March 11, 2004, presented evalu-

ations of fifteen HIV+ prisoners living in Dorms 6A, 6B, 7A, and 7B and five mortality reviews of prisoners who died in 2003. See Tabet 2003, 2004.

21. Tabet 2003, 15.

22. Ibid., 17.

23. Ibid.,18.

24. Deposition of Dr. Collette Simon taken before Maurice Lapidus, Commissioner of the Notary Republic, at 1200 Financial Center, Birmingham, AL, November 6, 2003, p. 22.

25. Ibid.

26. Tabet 2003, 190.

27. Ibid., 191.

28. See Hoover et al. 1993.

29. Tabet 2003, 194.

30. Deposition of Dr. Simon, November 6, 2003, at 29.

31. Typically, prisoner administrators either will declare they are doing the best they can or will minimize the scope of the problem. For an analysis of this phenomenon in New York, see von Zielbauer 2005a.

32. See Deposition of Dr. Simon, November 6, 2003, at 25, where Dr. Simon describes the need to only do "patient care."

33. See Liptak 2003, 17.

34. Dr. Simon is quite candid about the challenges of working for a for-profit health care provider. Specifically, she describes the reality of the company rejecting her requests for treatments outside of her area of expertise: "I've dealt with HMO's before [and] you have to be prepared for some rejection" (Deposition of Dr. Simon, November 6, 2003, at 46).

35. Ibid.

36. For an analysis documenting the crucial role prisoner activists play in obtaining compliance through aggressive education campaigns inside penal institutions, see Maddow 2001.

37. Richard 1986, 327.

38. Ibid.

39. Ibid.

40. This term comes from Dimaggio and Powell 1991. It is particularly useful for calling attention to how the institutional conditions at Limestone cannot be separated from Dr. Simon's choices as a physician. How "good people," such as Dr. Simon, are able to do the "dirty work" of the profoundly constrained environment of prison health care delivery has received considerable interest by sociologists studying other challenging organizational contexts. Diane Vaughan (1996, 36) succinctly explains this line of inquiry.

One of the enduring puzzles in the search for the causes of organizational misconduct is the question of "good" people and "dirty" work: how is it that people who are employed, have opportunities and education, and appear to have a lifetime record as law-abiding citizens can and do violate rules, regulations, and laws, doing harm in furtherance of organizational goals?

For other important discussions of organizational deviance, see Jackall 1988; H. Simon 1976; Weick 1979; March and Olsen 1979; Lindblom 1959.

41. See Jones 1993 for a compelling account of the institutional failures at the core of the Tuskegee syphilis experiment. For an excellent collection of essays on corporate and governmental deviance, see Ermann and Lundman 2001.

42. Vaughan 1996, 113.

43. Ibid., 100.

44. Monahan and Quinn 2006, 380.

45. Miller 1991, 10.

46. See Monahan and Quinn 2006.

47. See Gerber 2000 for a far-reaching account of the disabled veteran in history. For documentation of the dehumanization of traumatized Vietnam veterans, see Shay 1994; for the maltreatment of World War I veterans, see Moley 1966.

48. Gerber 2000, 78.

49. Priest and Hull 2007, A1.

50. See Cloud 2007.

51. Shay 1994, 4.

52. Quoted in Siegal 1998, 2.

53. Quoted in ibid., 2.

54. See Belkin 1999.

55. For two detailed studies demonstrating the devastating psychological effects of long-term isolation in Supermax prisons, see Haney 2003; Toch 2001.

56. Human Rights Watch, *Ill-Equipped: U.S. Prisons and Offenders with Mental Illness* (New York: Human Rights Watch, 2003), 153, http://www.hrw.org/reports/2003/usa1003/usa1003.pdf.

57. See "Position Statement of the American Association of Community Psychiatrists on Persons with Mental Illness Behind Bars," http://www.comm.psych.pitt.edu/finds/mibb.html.

CHAPTER 2

1. Oshinsky 1997.

2. D. McDonald 1999, 432.

3. Zahn and McBride 2000, 1A.

4. Ibid., 5.

5. Ludlow 2003, 1A.

6. Sward and Wallace 1994, A1.

7. See ibid., A4.

8. By July 2007, two federal judges issued orders to dramatically decrease California's prison population. The order has yet to be considered by the Ninth Circuit Court of Appeals. See Moore 2007.

9. Sillen 2006, E1.

10. Gerritt 2006.

11. Von Zielbauer 2005a, A1.

12. Paget 1988, 58.

13. Stoller 2003, 2264.

14. See Monahan and Quinn 2006 for an analysis of individual-level justifications focusing on "bad apples" as responsible for the scandal at Abu Ghraib prison.

15. See Eigenberg 1989 and 2000 for empirical studies of correctional officers' perceptions of prisoner rape and homosexuality. Both studies provide important insight into the complex and contradictory perceptions of officers that provide an important window into correctional officer subculture and what is behind an often uninformed, aggressive response to both aggressors and victims of homosexual rape behind bars. Eigenberg (2000, 430) observes:

> Consistent with prior research, most officers in this study indicated they would respond aggressively to any prohibitive acts whether they were consensual or coercive in nature . . . This finding is problematic because it may be impossible for officers to determine whether inmates are engaged in consensual or coercive acts merely by observing a sexual interaction . . . [W]hat appears on the surface to be consensual may, in fact, be coercive behavior.

See Nagel 1973 for a former prison official's account of the routine use of excessive force on the part of prison guards in one penal institution. See J. Mc-Donald 2007 for a very recent scandal involving prison guards who traded favors for sex from prisoners in Pennsylvania. For a discussion of the ethical dimensions and complexities of the subculture of correctional officers, see Stohr et al. 2000.

16. See Vaughn and Carroll 1998; Vaughn and Smith 1999.

17. Clear 1994, 4.

18. These figures are available on the bureau's Web site, at http://www.ojp.usdoj.gov/bjs/glance/incrt.htm.

19. This report is available on the Web site of the Sentencing Project, at http://www.sentencingproject.org/Admin%5CDocuments%5Cpublica tions%5Cinc_newfigures.pdf.

20. See Teeters 1955 for an account of Walnut Street Jail's struggle to overcome deplorable conditions, overcrowding, and contagious disease outbreaks.

21. See Gostin 1995 for a comprehensive history and review.

22. J. Simon 2007, 142.

23. See J. Simon 1997 for an analysis of the historical development of parole in California and the ways rehabilitation has given way to waste management.

24. See J. Simon 2007, 143. This program of mass incarceration was warmly embraced by George W. Bush's administration and Attorney General Ashcroft. Beyond its specific focus on toughening gun laws, Project Exile comprises a larger constellation of commitments that presents Americans with the option of obtaining more security for beleaguered urban cores by sending the young men of those communities into "exile."

25. Commenting on their own five-year field study of medical care in one U.S. jail in the 1990s, Vaughn and Smith (1999, 217) cogently observe: "The practice of penal harm medicine also fits the new penal managerialism or the new penology, whereby individual prisoners' rights are deemphasized and the efficient control of aggregate prisoner populations predominates. In this environment, it is acceptable to harm 'subhuman' prisoners."

26. D. McDonald 1999, 469.

27. Ibid., 471.

28. Schlesinger 2005, 93.

29. See Sered and Fernandopulle 2005.

30. See Robbins 1999 for a legal analysis that documents the deeply problematic mismatch between privatized health care and prison.

31. Robbins 1999, 235.

32. Quoted in Maddow 2001, 192.

33. Quoted in ibid.

34. See Hammett et al. 1995.

35. Names of ex-prisoners have been changed to preserve confidentiality.

36. Phone interview by Benjamin Fleury-Steiner, March 5, 2003.

37. Tamara Serwer, interview by Benjamin Fleury-Steiner, January 13, 2003.

38. Ibid. After numerous rounds of negotiation, Serwer ultimately was

able to convince the county to settle the case and make dramatic improvements to the quality of HIV care in the jail.

39. See Cook 2004 for a discussion of the reforms at Fulton County Jail. However, the positive changes were not to last. Fulton County Jail dramatically cut the number of staff and has since experienced dangerous overcrowding, with raw sewage spilling into some sections of the jail. See Cook 2006.

40. Alexander 2003, 70.

CHAPTER 3

1. Feeley 2003, 120.

2. See Greene 2002 and Hallet 2006 for detailed documentations of how the veritable floodgates of profit were opened to private prison companies.

3. See Sanger 2003.

4. Commenting on the flawed logic of the Reagan administration's plan to further privatize U.S. health care and cut public funds strategy, leading public health scholar Vicente Navarro (1984, 70) observed at the time: "Waste plus insufficient coverage are indeed the outcome of the 'free market' forces. Evidence from international comparisons shows that the problem is not too much government intervention but rather too little." See Navarro 1986, for a trenchant analysis of health care inequalities internationally and in the United States during the Reagan years.

5. See Wood 2003.

6. The *Newsweek* article ("Prohibition and Drugs") and Friedman's later observations on the failures of tough sentencing policies are available on the Web site of the Schaffer Library of Drug Policy, at http://www.druglibrary.org/special/friedman/milton_friedman.htm.

7. See Caldicott 2004 for a provocative analysis of the George W. Bush administration's massive investments in the nuclear defense industry.

8. Ronen Shamir (2004, 660) has written eloquently on the empty promises of "corporate social responsibility" in the context of a "neoliberal logic of altruistic social participation that is to be governed by goodwill alone."

9. See Melossi 1980, 20, for an especially important critique of the limits of Rusche and Kirchheimer's perspective for "capturing the inner structure of the prison institution, as a section of a broader bourgeois program"

10. Rusche and Kirchheimer 1939, 5.

11. See Garland 2001b and Gottschalk 2006.

12. Feeley 2003. Wendy Brown (2006, 698) clearly explains how neoconservatism and neoliberalism can operate together: "What we have in neoliberalism and neoconservatism, then, is a market-political rationality and a moral-political rationality, with a business model of the state in one case and

a theological model of the state in the other." This connection seems especially relevant for understanding how neoconservative co-optation of the moral high ground on law and order fits seamlessly into a massive, neoliberal "tough on crime" marketplace.

13. Wacquant 2001b, 404; see also Wacquant 2001b..

14. Western and Beckett 1999, 1053.

15. W. Brown 2006, 694.

16. Clear 1994. For a survey analysis documenting a far less punitive public, see Cullen, Fisher, and Applegate 2000.

17. Mauer and Chesney-Lind 2002. Megan Comfort (2008, 220) has described the shortcomings of the "invisible punishment" perspective of mass incarceration as overly criminal policy–oriented and without sufficient attention to "America's decrepit and fast-vanishing social-welfare state."

18. Ibid., 1–2.

19. Western 2006, 50. For other studies that find very little empirical support that recent crime drops are linked to mass incarceration policies, see Young and Brown 1993; Tonry 1995; Spelman 2000.

20. Gottschalk 2006, 75.

21. With regard to mass incarceration policies passed as part of America's war on drugs, Steiner (2001, 203) observes: "Investigating the War on Drugs reveals how criminal justice policies of the present are filtered through the lens of prevailing and pervasive inequalities. Indeed lawmaking is a highly contingent and dynamic process that can evoke divisive and often racist and chauvinistic stories of the past that lead to the revising of contemporary moralities and thus the implementation of racially and ethnically targeted anti-drug policies."

22. Glasser (2000, 723) states:

What we see, in effect, is that drug prohibition has become a replacement system for segregation. It has become a system of separating out, subjugating, imprisoning, and destroying substantial portions of a population based on skin color. And then you pick up the sociology journals, and they all are talking about the American family. And they all want to know, what happened to the black men? Where are they? They're dead in the streets. They're stopped on our highways. They're languishing in our prisons, and they can't vote. And all of that has to do, not with poverty by itself, but with government policy.

23. See Beckett 1997, 28–44, for an overview of the early politics of race, law, and order.

24. See Massing 2000 for a historical overview of modern-day U.S. policy on drug control. Massing persuasively shows how the more enlightened

Nixonian approach to drugs as a public health issue became more punitive by the end of the 1960s and has changed little ever since.

25. See Epstein 1977 for a history of Nixon's "war on heroin," as well as an earlier account of the racist application of early antidrug laws, such as the Harrison Act of 1914.

26. Byrd and Clayton 2002, 486. Commenting on the growing deterioration in the health status of blacks after 1980, leading sociologist of public health Nicolette Hart (1997, 109) observes, "This almost certainly reflects the increase of poverty sponsored by 'Reaganite' policies in the 1980s, demonstrating the sensitivity of longevity as a barometer of social and economic inequality."

27. See Cole 2000 for a trenchant account of how courts have not only acquiesced but played an active role in institutionalizing these assumptions into legal policies that invest in racial and class inequality.

28. See Steiner and Argothy 2001; Byrd and Clayton 2002.

29. Philadelphia assistant district attorney William Spade calls attention to the direct impact that the Bias incident had in the passage of the draconian hundred-to-one sentencing disparity between federal crack and cocaine cases. In a disturbing irony, it is likely that Bias did not die from an overdose of crack cocaine. Spade (1996, 1250) observes:

> Ironically, because the circumstances surrounding Bias's death were distorted by the media, the legislators who enacted the 1986 Act, as well as the American public, misunderstood the role that crack played in his death. Bias died of cocaine intoxication the day after he was the second player drafted in the National Basketball Association's 1986 college draft. At the time of his death, it was not known, outside a small group of people who had been with him, what method of cocaine ingestion he had used. Papers across the country nevertheless ran stories that quoted Maryland's Assistant Medical Examiner, Dr. Dennis Smyth, that Bias had died of "free-basing" cocaine. There were several other medical analyses of the probable method of cocaine ingestion. For instance, Dr. Yale Caplan, a toxicologist in the Maryland Medical Examiner's Office, said that a test of cocaine found in a vial at the scene "probably was not crack." Similarly, Maryland's Chief Medical Examiner, Dr. John Smialek, stated that evidence of cocaine residue in Bias's nasal passages suggested that Bias probably snorted cocaine. However, Dr. Smyth's statement received most of the coverage.

30. See Dvorak 2000 for an in-depth analysis of the policy debates surrounding the passage of the hundred-to-one disparity.

31. *Antidrug Abuse Act of 1986*, 99th Cong., 2d sess., *Congressional Record* 132 (September 26, 1986): S 26, 458.

32. In 1994, the Georgia General Assembly passed a "sentencing reform act" that enables a jury to impose life without parole for a second "serious violent felony." See Boreman 2001 for a detailed overview of the passage of the "two strikes" legislation in Georgia.

33. For example, the high-profile African American New York congressman Charles Rangel actively supported the hundred-to-one disparity, even going so far as to introduce a *New York Times* article depicting, as legal scholar Laura A. Wystma (1995, 505) observes, "crack's impending threat to civilized society." According to Wystma (504), the introduction of these sensationalized media accounts had racially explosive impact on legislators.

These stereotypical images undoubtedly influenced racial perceptions held by legislators concerning the "crack epidemic." The sensational reports fed white society's fear of the black male as a crack user and as a source of social disruption. The public was conditioned to think of crack users and pushers as the "enemy" responsible for increased violent crime. Consequently, the domestic enemy was distanced and devalued so that it became easy to forget that the "enemy" consisted of equal human beings. The prospect of crack spilling out into the white suburbs led legislators to instinctively punish black crack violators more harshly than their white, suburban, powder cocaine dealing counterparts. The ultimate outcome was the enactment of a draconian crack statute that levels exceedingly harsh penalties against its black violators as opposed to the weaker sentences imposed on white, cocaine-using infractors.

34. I have observed elsewhere (Fleury-Steiner 2002, 549): "Racial discourses constitute taken-for-granted understandings and practices. They serve as mechanisms of social control because they assert and instantiate differentiation but do not reveal the basis of those distinctions." See also Crenshaw 1995; Lipsitz 1998.

35. See Steiner 2001; Dvorak 2000; Wystma 1995.

36. Buckley 1986.

37. Perrow and Guillén 1990, 52.

38. C. Cohen 1999, 341.

39. Some commentators correctly call attention to the racially incendiary campaign speech Reagan made in August 1980 at Philadelphia, Mississippi, the site of the murders of three civil rights workers. In the speech, Reagan touted the need for a revitalized "states' rights." Such a speech reveals, at the very least, that Reagan attempted to play on the deeply seated racial fears of some Southern whites. See Marable 1991, 180.

40. Sen 2003, xvi.

41. See Farmer 2002.

42. The 2007 report, by Christopher Mumola, is available on the bureau's Web site, at http://www.ojp.usdoj.gov/bjs/pub/pdf/mcdsp04.pdf.

43. Stone 2005, 79.

44. Bertram et al. 1996, 37.

45. Schneider 1998, 433.

46. See Watters and Lewis 1990; Bluthenthal et al. 1997; Kral et al. 1998.

47. Day 1997, 3.

48. The report is available on the bureau's Web site, at http://www.ojp.usdoj.gov/bjs/glance/incrt.htm.

49. The report, by Judith Green and Kevin Pranis, is available online at http://www.justicestrategies.net/files/Alabama_Prison_Crisis_Oct_2005.pdf.

50. Although the reforms have restored some judicial discretion, New York judges are still only given prison as an option for even the lowest-level drug offenses. See Benjamin 2005.

51. See n. 49.

52. See Kirk A. Johnson, "What to Do about the Prison Problem: The Pros and Cons of Privatized Prisons in Alabama," 3, report of the Alabama Policy Institute, http://apcto.org/pdf/APIstudy.pdf.

53. Quoted in ibid.

54. Rothman [1980] 2002a, 426.

55. See the report "State Prison Expenditures, 2001," available on the Web site of the Bureau of Justice Statistics, at http://www.ojp.gov/bjs/pub/pdf/spe01.pdf.

56. The report is available on the Web site of the Alabama Department of Public Health, at http://www.adph.org/aids/assets/SurveillanceReport2005.pdf.

57. Levenson 2004, 25.

58. Ibid., 26.

59. See Sered and Fernandopulle 2005, 1–2.

60. Ibid.

61. D. McDonald 1999, 469.

62. For the effects of deindustrialization on the urban black poor, see Anderson 1990. For the anchoring effects of wealth inequality, see Oliver and Shapiro 1997. For the widespread marginalizing influences of racial segregation, see Massey and Denton 1993.

63. For a study of white flight in Atlanta and the politics that helped undermine black resistance to urban ghettoization, see Kruse 2005.

64. See B. M. Wilson 2000, 153.

65. Ibid.

66. See ibid., 154.

67. Jonathan Kozol, "Still Separate, Still Unequal: America's Educational Apartheid," *Harper's Magazine* 311, no. 1864 (September 1, 2005), available at http://www.mindfully.org/Reform/2005/American-Apartheid-Education1 sep05.htm (accessed March 2008).

68. Neubeck and Cazenave 2001, 12.

69. Sanger 2003, 5.

70. Drawing on both quantitative data from the 1991 National Race and Political Study and content analysis of forty-five years of media coverage, Martin Gilens (1999) finds powerful evidence of an entrenched racialization of welfare recipients as black, lazy, and abusers of the system.

71. Information on Alabama tax law and reform is made available by the Arise Citizens' Policy Project, a social and economic justice group. More detailed information can be found on the group's Web site, http://www.arisecit izens.org/.

72. This information comes from the organization's Web site, http://www.constitutionalreform.org/.

73. The ITEP report is available online at http://www.itepnet.org/ wp2000/text.pdf.

74. Maddow 2001, 191.

75. Davis 1999, L1.

76. Nicholson-Crotty 2004b, 46.

77. Ibid., 51–52.

78. Between 1995 and 1996, numerous new "tough on crime" laws aimed at curtailing prisoner rights were passed as part of the Republican's Contract with America, including the Violent Crime Control and Law Enforcement Improvement Act of 1995, the Taking Back Our Streets Act of 1995, the Violent Criminal Incarceration Act of 1995, the Stop Turning Out Prisoners Act, the Local Law Enforcement Enhancement Act of 1995, the Prison Litigation Reform Act of 1995, the Prison Conditions Litigation Reform Act, the Prisoner Lawsuit Efficiency Act of 1995, the Crime Prevention and Family Protection Act of 1996, and the Criminal Correction and Victim Assistance Act of 1996.

79. For studies of the distorted effects of "tort reform" rhetoric on the legal system, see Hans 2000 and Haltom and McCann 2004.

80. Schlanger 2003, 1620.

81. Ibid., 1586.

82. Ibid., 1589.

83. Schlanger (2003, 1,635) states:

Indeed, the National Association of Attorneys General pushed hard for state PLRAs, both before and after Congress passed the federal statute.

Largely as a result of this push, all but a few states now have some kind of system that specially regulates inmate access to state court.

84. Schlanger 2003, 1694.

85. *Prison Litigation Reform Act of 1995,* 104th Cong., 1st sess., *Congressional Record* 141 (September 27, 1995): S 14,413.

86. See Hill 2002 for an engrossing analysis of the sensationalist cases that elites employed in calling for the PLRA.

87. See Newman 1996.

88. Ibid., 521.

89. See ibid., 522.

90. Ibid.

91. See *Congressional Record* 141 (September 29, 1995): S 14,626.

92. This literature is too vast to review in detail here. For an overview of disturbing health care cases in Alabama, see Yackle 1989. For a small sampling of recent scandals from other states, see appendix B in the present study. For a former prisoner's account of the woefully inadequate health care at Attica, see Domino 2006. For a riveting account of the lack of adequate mental health care behind bars, see Kupers 2001. For a recent, wide-reaching documentation of health care problems facing incarcerated women, see Braithwaite, Arriola, and Newkirk 2006.

93. *Congressional Record* 141 (September 29, 1995): S 14,626.

94. See Farmer 2002 for a riveting account of the "criminalization" of tuberculosis at Attica. See Griswold 1999 for the recent chaos surrounding issues of overcrowding and maltreatment of tuberculosis in Fresno County jails in California. See Bidwell 1999 for a similar account of Los Angeles County jails.

95. See appendix B for an overview of fundamental institutional failures. See Herivel and Wright 2003, 168–210, for detailed stories of how private prison health providers have committed numerous, often dangerous mistakes in states around the country.

96. Although most institutions had medications available, there were likely many serious problems with actual access. See Siegal 1998. Moreover, as I make clear in the conclusion to the present study, some states require prisoners to participate in controversial drug trials before receiving medication. Even in this scenario, it has been discovered in one institution that when prisoners return from drug trials, prison guards often seize, out of security concerns, the samples of new medications that they bring with them. See Ward and Bishop 2001.

97. See Schlanger 2003, 1694.

98. Haney 1998, 32

99. See Ortega 1999.

100. Quoted in La Ganga and Richter 1996, A3.

CHAPTER 4

1. Ellen Barry, interview by Benjamin Fleury-Steiner, conducted March 21, 2003.

2. *Estelle v. Gamble* 429 U.S. 97 (1976), at 102–3. The quote "torture or a lingering death" comes from *In re Kemmler,* 136 U.S. 436 (1890), at 447; "unnecessary and wanton infliction of pain" is from *Gregg v. Georgia,* 428 U.S. 153 (1976), at 173.

3. Herman 1998, 1250–51.

4. See Sturm 1993 for an excellent overview.

5. See Feeley and Rubin 1998 for a comprehensive and balanced overview of the impact judicial action has had on prison conditions. Interestingly, despite all the positive procedural changes prisons have undergone in recent decades, Feeley and Rubin (378–79) conclude:

Most significant of all the courts never provided any real help with the single greatest problem facing prison administrators—the inmate population explosion . . . Cells designed for one person now hold two or three, school rooms and gymnasiums have been converted into dormitories, tent camps and trailer parks for inmates have sprouted in the prison yard, training and rehabilitation programs have been either overwhelmed with participants or restricted to small fractions of the eligible inmates, and prison officials have been compelled to shift from management to coping strategies.

6. Schlanger 2003, 2017.

7. See Greenberg 1994 for an autobiographical account of an LDF lawyer who worked on such cases from the late 1940s through the civil rights movement era of the 1960s.

8. See Yackle 1989 for perhaps the most concise overview of Judge Johnson's developing judicial approach to the Alabama prison cases.

9. *Newman v. Alabama,* 559 F.2d 283 (5th Cir. 1977), at 19.

10. Sturm 1993, 642.

11. *Newman v. Alabama,* at 13.

12. Yackle 1989, 260.

13. Feeley and Rubin 1998, 375.

14. Ibid.

15. Scott 1990. While Scott's work falls into the category of "new social movements" (NSM) theory (see Calhoun 1993 for an overview and critique of the early roots of NSM), his work is particularly important as one of the first

works to advocate for a more direct embrace of the sociopolitical context of social movement activism. By contrast to NSM's traditionally more macro focus on the influence of structural conditions on mobilization, Scott calls for a far more direct approach to the analysis of how movement ideology is constituted as social action. For a more exhaustive critique of NSM, See Pichardo 1997.

16. Maddow 2001, 7.

17. But Maddow (2001, 9) herself concedes:

The HIV/AIDS movement is stratified; it has more enthusiastically defined community expertise and resisted coercive measures against people with HIV/AIDS who are gay but otherwise relatively socially advantaged, than it has among other populations disproportionately affected by the epidemic, including prisoners. Prisoners with HIV/AIDS and their advocates have thus faced punishing, stigmatizing measures with only half-hearted support from the outside HIV/AIDS movement, but even that half-hearted effort stands in stark contrast to the persistent division between health care provision inside and outside of prisons.

18. Stockdill 2003, 89–90.

19. Morris's own research (1984, 1992) on the civil rights movement is particularly illuminating in the way that it problematizes activist ideology as multiple and often fragmented. Morris (1992, 364) notes that "those oppressed by one system of domination may in fact enjoy a position of privilege and power in another." See also Stoller 1998.

20. Barry 2000, 172.

21. Maddow (2001, 206) reports, "By 2000, care for prisoners with HIV/AIDS at Vacaville would be widely considered among prison HIV/AIDS advocates to be among the best, if not the best, in the country." But Vacaville has had its share of recent institutional crises, including delayed transfers of critically ill patients that resulted in preventable death (see Sillen 2006).

22. Ellen Barry, interview by the author, March 21, 2003.

23. For a fuller account of the *Shumate* support coalition, see Maddow 2001, 116–17.

24. See ibid.

25. See Stoller 2001.

26. Ibid., 95.

27. In my March 21, 2003, interview with her, leading prisoner rights activist Ellen Barry argues:

Since the PLRA, one of the things that we find most troubling is how difficult it is for prisoners to clear the administrative appeals hurdles. That has stopped a whole lot of activism in its tracks. We have tracked a large number of cases. We had, I would say, comparable, factual cases coming up on neglect and abuses, lack of adequate medical care. But we couldn't get anyone to clear the administrative hurdles because of a whole series of things. I think that corrections early on got it, stopped the administrative appeals and stop litigation . . . There were so many appeals ripped up right in your face, "You have no right to this, (rip, rip) I am throwing it away."

28. Edelman 1992, 1436. For other studies of the interplay between legal and institutional change, see L. Jacobs 2007; Taylor 2006; Albiston 2006; Edelman, Erlanger, and Lande 1993.

29. To preserve confidentiality, all names are changed.

30. This account and the other accounts presented in the remainder of this chapter come from interviews previously published in Fleury-Steiner and Hodge 2006, 159–78. They are selected from twenty-five interviews that were conducted with advocates who work in post-PLRA prisons and jails from across the United States. The interviews were conducted between October and December of 2004. For clarity of presentation, respondents' quotes were edited for style.

31. Under the Violent Crime Control and Law Enforcement Act of 1994, a remarkable $7.9 billion was authorized by Congress for prison construction. See Masci 1994, 2490.

32. Before it was dramatically amended by the PLRA, CRIPA put strict requirements on prisons to utilize effective administrative remedies when dealing with prisoner complaints.

33. *Civil Rights of Institutionalized Persons Act, U.S. Code* 42 (1980), Section A1.

34. A recent report by the New York State Senate Democratic Task Force on Criminal Justice Reform reveals that approximately fifty-five hundred prisoners in New York State are currently being held in SHUs. Once inside, prisoners are held under twenty-three-hour lockdown (see Parenti 2000).

35. Human Rights Watch, *Ill-Equipped: U.S. Prisons and Offenders with Mental Illness* (New York: Human Rights Watch, 2003), 153, http://www.hrw.org/reports/2003/usa1003/usa1003.pdf..

CHAPTER 5

1. Unless otherwise noted, all quotes from SCHR personnel are taken from interviews by the author that took place on March 4–5, 2003.

2. See Crowder 2006.

3. Ibid., 17A.

4. Ibid.

5. Ibid., 18A

6. See Feeley and Swearingen 2004.

7. Crowder 2006, 18A.

8. Ibid.

9. Ibid.

10. See Walzer 2004 for a detailed scientific overview of the infection.

11. See Sturm 1993.

12. Ibid., 648.

13. For a comprehensive overview of the legality of HIV+ prisoners' rights, see Haas 1993.

14. See *Harris v. Thigpen,* 941 F.2d (11th Cir. 1991) 126 F.3d (11th Civ. 1997); *Onishea v. Hopper* 1999; *Davis v. Hopper,* cert. denied, 120 U.S. 93 (2000).

15. See Greenhouse 2000.

16. Sturm 1993, 644.

17. For example, Maddow and ACLU activists convinced Mississippi to open educational and drug treatment programs to HIV+ prisoners in the state. See Wagster 2001 for coverage of the change in the state.

18. Maddow 2001, 327.

19. See Dimaggio and Powell 1991. See Rogers-Dillon and Skretny 1999 for an analysis of how the media has been influential in fostering a legitimacy imperative in the administering of Florida's recent welfare reform—what the authors call a "success imperative."

20. Such a strategy was first honed five years prior to the *Leatherwood* litigation, in the successful class action case *Shumate v. Wilson,* which focused on California's HIV+ prison population. As briefly discussed in previous sections, the *Shumate* case was considered by many prisoner rights attorneys and activists around the United States to be a powerful catalyst not only for taking on the HIV and AIDS crisis behind bars but for reinvigorating the broader struggle against the excesses of mass incarceration and a dramatic narrowing of prisoner rights in the United States. Beyond the legal victory of securing stronger privacy rights for HIV+ prisoners in California, *Shumate* demonstrated something important to a community that had felt the sting of the increasingly "tough on crime" forces of the last decade. It became clear that the new approach to prisoner conditions and health care issues would have to depend on broad coalitions of lawyers, medical experts, activists, and especially former prisoners. What made *Shumate* successful was its aggressive approach to prisoner advocacy that highlighted prisoner concerns, educating the public to the horrors of mass incarceration, and conceiving of litigation as a tool of last resort.

21. See Maddow 2001.

22. See http://www.criticalresistance.org/.

23. The "No Lost Causes" conference was held on June 17, 2000. The event's final session described the overriding objective.

After more than two decades of concerted efforts by prisoners' advocates to protect the rights of HIV positive prisoners, many of the most egregious cases remain unchanged and unresolved. This session will look at the connections necessary for sustained, effective action campaigns. Possible topics include: how to bring prison issues to the attention of local legislators; building relationships between churches, AIDS service organizations and groups representing people of color; how and when to pitch a story to local media; bringing national attention to bear on local issues.

24. Jackie Walker, interview by the author, March 24, 2003.

25. The first step of Maddow and longtime NPP investigator Jackie Walker was to contact HIV+ prisoners in both Mississippi and Alabama. Mississippi prisoners described to them the woefully inadequate care they were receiving and their strong desire to have access to prison programs. Remarkably, not only did Maddow, Walker, and other advocates persuade Mississippi and Alabama corrections officials to attend the "No Lost Causes" conference, but they miraculously convinced Mississippi officials that it was in their best interest to both end segregating HIV+ prisoners from the general public and allow them to participate in vital education and job programs.

Walker's many years of prisoner advocacy in Alabama had made her all too aware of how injustice, inhumanity, and institutional inertia ruled prison governance in the state. Likewise, Elizabeth Alexander, current NPP director and lead attorney in the ACLU's early AIDS/HIV cases, was well aware, as she puts it during an interview with the author on April 9, 2003, of "how completely out of touch the judges down there were about HIV and AIDS." She adds, "I mean, they were worried that they could be infected by eating peanut butter." Interviews Maddow and Walker conducted with Alabama's current HIV+ population revealed lasting fears of a continued and potentially dangerous antipathy on the part of the general population and prison staff. It was clear to Maddow and Walker that HIV + prisoners wanted access to prison programs. However, Alabama's HIV+ prison population uniformly opposed being reintegrated back into the general population. Maddow explains: "They had said that because this segregation program had been going on for nearly seventeen years, they were convinced that ending it would result in a violent backlash against them. So, it wasn't that they didn't want to stay in this segregated hellhole out of choice; they simply feared for their very lives, and we were going to respect those wishes" (interview by the author, May 14, 2003).

26. Jackie Walker, interview by the author, March 3, 2003.

27. *Leatherwood v. Campbell,* No. CV-02-BE-2812-W (N.D. Ala., June 3, 2004), 5. The complete opinion is available on SCHR's Web site, at http://www.schr.org/prisonsjails/press%20releases/Magistrate%20Report%20Recommendation.pdf.

28. Ibid., 5–6.

29. Ibid., 7–8.

CHAPTER 6

1. Whenever possible in this chapter, in order to provide additional information on the final days of Limestone prisoners' lives as well as any further details that help to humanize them beyond the identity of "dying prisoner," I turn to interviews that *Birmingham News* reporter Carla Crowder conducted with former prisoners who knew the prisoner identified. The interviews took place on July 25, 2006. Unless otherwise noted, all quotes with former prisoners are taken from these interviews.

2. Both of the report's volumes are available on SCHR's Web site, at http://www.schr.org/prisonsjails/news/Limestone/Limestone.html.

3. See Crowder 2006 and von Zielbauer 2005b for two noteworthy exceptions.

4. See Crowder 2006.

5. See B. McEwen 2005.

6. Shorey 2003.

7. Tabet 2003, 18.

8. See Crowder 2006, 17A.

9. Foucault [1975] 1995, 198.

10. Stoller 2003, 2265.

11. See Crowder 2006, 17A.

12. See ibid.

13. See Byrd and Clayton 2002; Sered and Fernandopulle 2005. See Kim et al. 2000 for a remarkable volume of case studies that document health care deprivation from around the world.

14. Stoller 2003, 2271.

15. Sered and Fernandopulle 2005, 215–16.

16. Wilson Rogers (name changed), interview by Carla Crowder, July 25, 2006.

17. Tabet 2003, 115.

18. Ibid.

19. Wilson Rogers (name changed), interview by Carla Crowder, July 25, 2006.

20. For fact sheets on diabetes, see http://www.diabetes.org.

21. Tabet 2003, 133.

22. Quoted in ibid., 100.

23. Quoted in ibid.

24. Quoted in ibid.

25. Ibid.

26. Ibid., 102.

27. A person's normal T cell count is between five hundred and fifteen hundred cells. See Michael and Kim 1999 for a detailed overview of HIV and the development of medical protocols for treating the virus.

28. Stoller 2003, 2268.

29. See Crowder 2006.

30. Tabet 2003, 147.

31. For extensive documentation of inadequate mental health services in the nation's penal institutions, see Human Rights Watch, *Ill-Equipped: U.S. Prisons and Offenders with Mental Illness* (New York: Human Rights Watch, 2003), 1, http://www.hrw.org/reports/2003/usa1003/usa1003.pdf. The report states:

> Somewhere between two and three hundred thousand men and women in U.S. prisons suffer from mental disorders, including such serious illnesses as schizophrenia, bipolar disorder, and major depression. An estimated seventy thousand are psychotic on any given day. Yet across the nation, many prison mental health services are woefully deficient, crippled by understaffing, insufficient facilities, and limited programs.

32. Septra is an inexpensive antibiotic used to treat PCP. Additional information is available online at http://www.drugs.com/cons/septra.html.

33. Tabet 2003, 89.

34. Ibid., 178.

35. See George Smith 2000, 182. See the rest of Smith's 2000 article for a discussion of the legal and social dimensions of the debate over humane assistance in end-of-life cases.

36. Tabet 2003, 186.

37. Ibid., 187.

38. Ibid., 188.

39. See the foundation's statement quoted earlier in this chapter and its Web site, http://www.americanhospice.org/.

40. Tabet 2003, 91.

41. Stoller 2003, 2270. Beyond "alternative spaces of care," it is perhaps more accurate to view these instances as evidence of a perverse "carceral community" that keeps uninsured HIV+ prisoners "enmeshed in and dependent on the criminal justice system as they attempt to create a safe, healthy and sustainable existence." See Comfort 2008, 197.

42. Tabet 2004, 56.

43. Quoted in Crowder 2006, A17.

44. Quoted in ibid., A17.

45. See Whitman 1990.

46. See *Harris v. Thigpen,* 941 F.2d (11th Cir. 1991).

47. Vaughn and Smith 1999, 178, citing T. M. Brown 1987, 156.

48. Peet 2004b, 3.

49. Ludlow 2003, 1A.

50. Quoted in Wedge 2001, 8.

51. McLachlin and Pacenti 2004, 1A.

52. Von Zielbauer 2005a, A1.

53. Oswald 1999.

CONCLUSION

1. See Tabet 2004, 9.

2. Ibid., 8.

3. Ibid., 43.

4. Ibid., 43.

5. Quote from SCHR's Web site, at http://www.schr.org/prisonsjails/news/Limestone/Limestone.html, where more details are available.

6. Von Zielbauer 2005b, A11.

7. Ibid.

8. Perrucci et al. 1980, 151.

9. Von Zielbauer 2005b, A12.

10. Monahan and Quinn 2006, 380.

11. Vaughn and Smith 1999, 219.

12. Zahn and McBride 2000, 1A.

13. See Nicholson-Crotty 2004a for a state-level analysis that demonstrates a significant linkage between low state prison expenditures and high prison populations. See Stucky, Heimer, and Lang 2007, 115, for an empirical analysis of state-level prison spending data that highlights "the underlying logic linking effects of party politics, racial threat, and state fiscal concerns."

14. Jacobson 2006.

15. See Wood and Dunaway 2003.

16. For a trenchant analysis of the influence of victim rights organizations

and other, less obvious activist groups (e.g., women's rights activists campaigning for tougher sentences for domestic violence), see Gottschalk 2006. See Zimring, Hawkins, and Kamin 2003 for a case study of the influence of victim rights groups, the NRA, and the corrections officer union in helping to pass California's "three strikes and you're out" laws.

17. Wood and Dunaway 2003, 150.

18. In February 2007, Superior Court judge Gail D. Ohanesian declared Schwarzenegger's "prisoner transfer" plan illegal. See Warren 2007.

19. Skolnick 1999. In an analysis of Skolnick's report, Rachel Maddow (2001, 195) summarizes the widespread problem of incompetent doctors currently working in penal settings in both Alabama and Missouri.

The director of mental health services in Alabama prisons was hired by Correctional Medical Services, Inc. (CMS) despite the fact that he had twice lost his medical license in other states due to sexual misconduct with both professional colleagues and patients . . . [T]he combination of recruitment difficulties in prison health and the enthusiastic lobbying of private companies has carved out a niche in which disciplined physicians have found a "last resort" to practice medicine . . . In Missouri, nine of the thirty-five physicians employed by CMS have been disciplined by medical authorities—a rate 10 times the national average.

20. Hornblum 1999.

21. Quoted in ibid.

22. See Urbina 2006.

23. Ward and Bishop 2001.

24. Ibid.

25. See Hammett, Roberts, and Kennedy 2001 for an excellent overview of the challenges to reentry for chronically ill prisoners.

26. See the Sentencing Project's 2004 report "State Rates of Incarceration by Race," http://www.sentencingproject.org/Admin/Documents/publications/rd_staterates.pdf.

27. For empirical analyses that show how state's with high levels of incarceration are far less concerned with prison conditions, as evidenced in dramatically lower spending levels, see Nicholson-Crotty 2004a; Stucky, Heimer, and Lang 2007.

28. See Mooney 1994.

29. See the report "State Prison Expenditures, 2001," available on the Web site of the Bureau of Justice Statistics, at http://www.ojp.gov/bjs/pub/pdf/spe01.pdf.

30. See Sillen 2006, E1.

31. See Sward and Wallace 1994.

32. See Williams and Parra 2005 for one article in the series.

33. See Sloop 1996.

34. According to a recent report from the Bureau of Justice Statistics, entitled "Medical Causes of Deaths in State Prison, 2001–2004," DICRA uncovered fifty-five additional AIDS-related deaths in 2001 and sixty-eight in 2002. But it is not clear how thorough prison reporting systems actually are. Indeed, the report's findings cast further doubt on the reliability of prisoner death statistics. Moreover, it is unclear whether DICRA will lead to dissemination of more qualitative related data concerning prisoner deaths. The 2007 report, by Christopher Mumola, is available on the bureau's Web site, at http://www.ojp.usdoj.gov/bjs/pub/pdf/mcdsp04.pdf.

35. To date, there are no clean-needle programs in U.S. penal institutions. Condoms are available in only six U.S. jails or prison systems (in Vermont, Mississippi, San Francisco, Dallas, Philadelphia, and New York City). See Hammett et al. 1995, 49.

36. An executive summary of the report is available on the NCCHC Web site, at http://www.ncchc.org/stbr/Volume1/ExecutiveSummary.pdf.

37. The quote is from chapter 7 of the report, available at http://www.ncchc.org/stbr/Volume1/Chapter7.pdf.

38. Nicholson-Crotty and Nicholson-Crotty 2004, 250.

39. Ibid., 251.

40. Ibid., 254.

41. Feeley and Swearingen 2004, 474.

42. For a powerful analysis documenting the effects of racialized state policy in maintaining cavernous wealth inequalities in the United States, see Oliver and Shapiro 1997. See Johnson 2006 for a provocative analysis of how the ideology of meritocracy and the "American dream" keeps many Americans in the dark about deepening inequalities in wealth and education.

43. Western, Pettit, and Guetzkow 2002, 178–79. Another devastating consequence of mass incarceration has been the draconian laws that impose a lifetime ban on public housing and welfare benefits for convicted drug offenders. Gwen Rubinstein and Debbie Mukamal (2002, 39) observe: "Two recently enacted policies driven by stigma and 'tough' on drugs rhetoric make it particularly difficult for low-income people with drug problems to afford treatment and basic necessities and to find safe and sober housing so they can successfully reintegrate back into community, live drug- and crime-free, and provide for themselves and their families."

44. Farmer 2003; Feeley and Swearingen 2004, 474.

45. J. Simon 2007, 21.

46. Farmer 2003, 180. Hepatitis C is a disease of the liver caused by the

Hepatitis C virus (HCV). Like HIV, HCV is a blood-borne virus that attacks and kills liver cells where it multiplies. Talvi (2003, 181) reports: "The nation's prisons are now harboring the highest concentrations of hepatitis C in the country. From state to state, from 20 to 60 percent of the current national prison population is believed to harbor the virus."

47. See *NIH Consensus Statement on Management of Hepatitis C: 2002,* NIH Consensus and State-of-the-Science Statements vol. 19, no. 3 (Bethesda, MD: National Institutes of Health, 2002), 9, http://consensus.nih.gov/2002/2002HepatitisC2002116PDF.pdf.

48. J. Simon 2007, 21.

49. Garland 2001a.

50. Ibid.; Rothman [1980] 2002a.

51. Byrd and Clayton 2002, 480–81.

52. Ibid., 481.

53. See Salmon 1990 for a discussion of the coining of the term in 1967.

54. Byrd and Clayton 2002, 489.

55. Ibid., 525–28.

56. Sered and Fernandopulle 2005, 6.

57. Ibid., 19.

58. Byrd and Clayton (2002, 484) observe:

Despite the initiation and perpetuation of policies that were counterproductive to the public's health; the emergence of unwholesome health system trends, policies, and practices; and the misuse and occasional abuse of publicly funded health resources, the public health community was virtually starved of essential funding and rendered almost silent.

59. See Horne 2006 for perhaps the most insightful account of Hurricane Katrina yet to be written.

60. O'Reilly's online rant "Katrina and the Poor" attests to his aggressive denial of America's continued failures to address centuries of entrenched racial oppression. The full article is available at http://www.billoreilly.com. Nowhere in the article do we learn about the making of the racial ghetto vis-à-vis lynchings and the burning of black-owned businesses by white supremacists in New Orleans well into the 1950s, the racist banking and real estate practices that remain an ever-present means for strengthening the color line, nor the Reagan administration's unprecedented gutting of funds for public health and other vital services needed by the nation's most racially aggrieved communities. Instead, the focus of O'Reilly's "Katrina and the Poor" is on America's so-called equal playing field and the color-blind racism (see Bonilla-Silva 2003) of blame that traffics in the fantasy world of "equality of opportunity" and "individual responsibility." O'Reilly writes:

The racial hustlers and far-left demagogues continue to sell victimization to Americans living in the poor precincts. The poverty pimps can't blame the establishment fast enough for ghettos and deprivation and even hurricanes. But you rarely hear the words "personal responsibility" when it comes to attacking the poverty problem.

61. The report is available online at http://www.gao.gov/new.items/do6403t.pdf.

62. All quotes from Cynthia Chandler are from an interview conducted by the author on March 28, 2003.

EPILOGUE

1. Interviews conducted by Carla Crowder, July 25, 2006.
2. See http://www.fellowshiphouse.org/.
3. The 2007 report, by Christopher Mumola, is available on the bureau's Web site, at http://www.ojp.usdoj.gov/bjs/pub/pdf/mcdsp04.pdf.
4. Scott Shane (2007, 14) reports that a recent panel headed by two former secretaries of the U.S. Army concluded that "the current system for assessing soldiers' disabilities is extremely cumbersome, inconsistent, and confusing," saying it must be "completely overhauled."
5. Rusche and Kirchheimer [1968] 1939, 207.

APPENDIX B

1. Silverman 1996.
2. Ward and Bishop 2001.
3. Ibid.
4. See Shurley and Smith 2003.
5. Fries 2007.
6. Prendergrast 1999.
7. Burton 1997.
8. See Associated Press 2005.
9. Quoted in Raynou 2003.
10. Quoted in Bauer 2000.
11. Greg Smith 1999.
12. Quoted in Peet 2004a, 1.
13. Quoted in Sentementes 2007, 5B.

REFERENCES

Acton, Andy. 2000. "Quarantined: Special Unit 16." *Birmingham Post-Herald,* August 26, A1–A5.

Albertini, William Oliver, Jr. 2004. "Catching Discourse: Contagion, Narrative, and U.S. Cultures at Century's End." PhD diss., University of Virginia.

Albiston, Catherine R. 2006. "Legal Consciousness and Workplace Rights." In *The New Civil Rights Research: A Constitutive Approach,* ed. Benjamin Fleury-Steiner and Laura-Beth Nielsen. Burlington, VT: Ashgate.

Alexander, Elizabeth. 2003. "Private Prisons and Health Care: The HMO from Hell." In *Capitalist Punishment: Prison Privatization and Human Rights,* ed. Andrew Coyle, Allison Campbell, and Rodney Neufeld. Atlanta: Clarity.

Anderson, Elijah. 1990. *Streetwise: Race, Class, and Change in an Urban Community.* Chicago: University of Chicago Press.

Associated Press. 2005. "State Investigating City Jails Health Care Provider." May 11.

Barker, Vanessa. 2006. "The Politics of Punishing: A State Governance Theory of American Imprisonment Variation." *Punishment and Society* 8:5–32.

Barry, Ellen. 2000. "Women Prisoners on the Cutting Edge: The Activist Women's Prisoners' Rights Movement." *Social Justice* 27:168–75.

Bauer, Scott. 2000. "State Prison's Medical Care in Disrepair." Associated Press, June 27.

Beckett, Katherine. 1997. *Making Crime Pay: Law and Order in Contemporary American Politics.* New York: Oxford University Press.

Belkin, Lisa. 1999. "A Brutal Cure." *New York Times,* May 30, 34–44.

Benjamin, Elizabeth. 2005. "Drug Law Changes Send Few to Freedom." *Times Union* (Albany, NY) December 15, A1.

Bertram, Eva, Morris J. Blachman, Kenneth Sharpe, and Peter Andreas. 1996. *Drug War Politics: The Price of Denial.* Berkeley: University of California Press.

Bidwell, Carol. 1999. "Waging the War against TB: Health Workers Keep on Fighting Deadly Malady." *Los Angeles Daily News,* April 19, 1–5.

Bluthenthal, Ricky N., Alex Kral, Jennifer Lovrick, and John K. Watters. 1997. "Impact of Law Enforcement on Syringe Exchange Programs." *Medical Anthropology* 18:61–83.

Bonilla-Silva, Eduardo. 2003. *Racism without Racists: Color-Blind Racism and the Persistence of Racial Inequality in America.* New York: Rowman and Littlefield.

Boreman, Brian D. 2001. "Mandatory Minimum Sentencing Survives Separation of Power Attacks, Remaining a Viable Option for the Legislature in Its War on Crime." *Georgia State University Law Review* 17:637–52.

Braithwaite, Ronald L., Kimberly Jacob Arriola, and Cassandra Newkirk. 2006. *Health Issues among Incarcerated Women.* Piscataway, NJ: Rutgers University Press.

Brown, T. M. 1987. "Doctors in Extremity." *Law, Medicine, and Health Care* 15:156–59.

Brown, Wendy. 2006. "American Nightmare: Neoliberalism, Neoconservatism, and De-Democratization." *Political Theory* 34:690–714.

Buckley, William F. 1986. "Crucial Steps in Combating the AIDS Epidemic; Identify All the Carriers." *New York Times*, March 18, Op-Ed.

Burawoy, Michael. 1998. "The Extended Case Method." *Sociological Theory* 16:4–33.

Burton, Greg. 1997. "Prison Health Care in Handcuffs." *Salt Lake Tribune*, October 26, C1–C3.

Byrd, W. Michael, and Linda A. Clayton. 2002. *An American Health Dilemma.* Vol. 2, *Race, Medicine, and Health Care in the United States, 1900–2000.* New York: Routledge.

Caldicott, Helen. 2004. *The New Nuclear Danger: George W. Bush's Military-Industrial Complex.* Rev. ed. New York: New Press.

Calhoun, Craig. 1993. "'New Social Movements' of the Early Nineteenth Century." *Social Science History* 17:385–427.

Clear, Todd R. 1994. *Harm in American Penology: Offenders, Victims, and Their Communities.* Albany: State University of New York Press.

Clemmer, Donald. 1940. *The Prison Community.* New York: Holt, Rinehart, and Winston.

Cloud, David S. 2007. "Army Secretary Ousted in Furor over Hospital Care." *New York Times*, March 2, 1–2.

Cohen, Cathy J. 1999. *The Boundaries of Blackness: AIDS and the Breakdown of Black Politics.* Chicago: University of Chicago Press.

Cohen, Stanley. 1985. *Visions of Social Control: Crime, Punishment, and Classification.* Cambridge, UK: Polity.

Cole, David. 2000. *No Equal Justice: Race and Class in the American Criminal Justice System.* New York: New Press.

Comfort, Megan L. 2002. "'Papa's House': The Prison as Domestic and Social Satellite." *Ethnography* 3:467–99.

Comfort, Megan L. 2008. *Doing Time Together: Love and Family in the Shadow of the Prison.* Chicago: University of Chicago Press.

Cook, Rhonda. 2004. "Fulton Jail Still Deficient." *Atlanta Journal-Constitution,* September 17, 1D.

Cook, Rhonda. 2006. "Sewage Spill Worsen Fulton Jail Crowding." *Atlanta Journal-Constitution,* April 21.

Crenshaw, Kimberle. 1995. "Mapping the Margins: Intersectionality, Identity Politics, and Violence against Women." In *After Identity,* ed. Dan Danielsen and Karen Engle. New York: Routledge.

Crowder, Carla. 2002. "Inmates' Medical Services Decried Lawsuit: Women's Care So Bad Some Pull Own Teeth, Others Denied Medication." *Birmingham News,* December 18, 1–3.

Crowder, Carla. 2003. "Jail Contractor to Treat Hepatitis C." *Birmingham News,* November 2, 1–3.

Crowder, Carla. 2004. "Judge: Prison's Care Violated Rights of HIV-Infected Inmates." *Birmingham News,* June 8, 1–3.

Crowder, Carla. 2005. "Ex-prisoner's Medical Woes Linger, Fester." *Birmingham News,* January 17, 1A–8A.

Crowder, Carla. 2006. "Prison Medical Failures Seen in Suit." *Birmingham News,* July 9, 17A–22A.

Cullen, Francis T., Bonnie S. Fisher, and Brandon K. Applegate. 2000. "Public Opinion about Punishment and Corrections." *Crime and Justice* 27:1–79.

Davis, Maia. 1999. "Change Sought in Inmate Health Care; Sheriff Wants Private Contractor Out." *(Bergen County, NJ) Record,* July 28, L1–L4.

Day, Dawn. 1997. *Health Emergency.* Princeton, NJ: Dogwood Center.

Dimaggio, Paul J., and Walter W. Powell. 1991. *The New Institutionalism in Organizational Analysis.* Chicago: University of Chicago Press.

Domino, John. 2006. *Attica: A Survivor's Story.* Longwood, FL: Xulon.

Dvorak, Richard. 2000. "Cracking the Code: 'De-Coding' Colorblind Slurs during the Congressional Crack Cocaine Debates." *Michigan Journal of Race and Law* 5:611–63.

Edelman, Lauren B. 1992. "Legal Ambiguity and Symbolic Structures: Organizational Mediation of Civil Rights Law." *American Journal of Sociology* 97:1531–76.

Edelman, Lauren B., Howard S. Erlanger, and John Lande. 1993. "Internal Dispute Resolution: The Transformation of Civil Rights in the Workplace." *Law and Society Review* 27:497–534.

Eigenberg, Helen. 1989. "Male Rape: An Empirical Examination of Correctional Officers' Attitudes toward Rape in Prison." *Prison Journal* 69: 39–56.

Eigenberg, Helen. 2000. "Correctional Officers and Their Perceptions of Homosexuality, Rape, and Prostitution in Male Prisoners." *Prison Journal* 80:415–33.

Epstein, Edward. 1977. *Agency of Fear: Opiates and Political Power in America.* New York: Putnam.

Ermann, M. David, and Richard J. Lundman. 2001. *Corporate and Governmental Deviance: Problems of Organizational Behavior in Contemporary Society.* New York: Oxford University Press.

Farmer, Paul. 2002. "The House of the Dead: Tuberculosis and Incarceration." In *Invisible Punishment: The Collateral Consequences of Mass Imprisonment,* ed. Marc Mauer and Meda Chesney-Lind. New York: New Press.

Farmer, Paul. 2003. *Pathologies of Power: Health, Human Rights, and the New War on the Poor.* Berkeley: University of California Press.

Feeley, Malcolm M. 2003. "Crime, Social Order, and Neo-conservative Politics." *Theoretical Criminology* 7:111–30.

Feeley, Malcolm M., and Edward L. Rubin. 1998. *Judicial Policy Making and the Modern State: How the Courts Reformed America's Prisons.* New York: Cambridge University Press.

Feeley, Malcolm M., and Van Swearingen. 2004. "The Prison Conditions Cases and the Bureaucratization of American Corrections: Influences, Impacts, and Implications." *Pace Law Review* 24:433–74.

Fleury-Steiner, Benjamin. 2002. "Narratives of the Death Sentence: Toward a Theory of Legal Narrativity." *Law and Society Review* 36:549–74.

Fleury-Steiner, Benjamin, and Jessica Hodge. 2006. "Keeping Rights Alive: The Struggle for HIV-Infected Prisoners." In *The New Civil Rights Research: A Constitutive Approach,* ed. Benjamin Fleury-Steiner and Laura-Beth Nielsen. Burlington, VT: Ashgate.

Foucault, Michel. [1975] 1995. *Discipline and Punish: The Birth of the Prison.* Reprint, New York: Vintage.

Friedman, Milton. 1962. *Capitalism and Freedom.* Chicago: University of Chicago Press.

Fries, Jacob H. 2007. "Burden on the Block." *St. Petersburg Times,* January 14, 1A–10A.

Garland, David. 2001a. *The Culture of Control: Crime and Social Order in Contemporary Society.* Chicago: University of Chicago Press.

Garland, David. 2001b. *Mass Imprisonment: Social Causes and Consequences.* London: Sage.

Gerber, David. 2000. *Disabled Veterans in History.* Ann Arbor: University of Michigan Press.

Gerritt, Jeff. 2006. "Needless Death Sentence: Level of Care in State Prisons Is Putting Health of Inmates at Risk." *Detroit Free Press,* June 19, 1–5.

Gilens, Martin. 1999. *Why Americans Hate Welfare: Race, Media, and the Politics of Antipoverity Policy.* Chicago: University of Chicago Press.

Gilman, Sander L. 1987. "AIDS and Syphilis: The Iconography of Disease." *AIDS: Cultural Analysis/Cultural Activism* 43:87–107.

Glasser, Ira. 2000. "American Drug Laws: The New Jim Crow." *Albany Law Review* 63:703–24.

Goffman, Erving. 1961. *Asylums: Essays on the Social Situation of Mental Patients and Other Inmates.* New York: Penguin.

Goifman, Kiko. 2002. "Killing Time in the Brazilian Slammer." *Ethnography* 3:436–41.

Gostin, Lawrence O. 1995. "The Resurgent Tuberculosis Epidemic in the Era of AIDS: Reflections on Public Health, Law, and Society." *Maryland Law Review* 54:4–131.

Gottschalk, Marie. 2006. *The Prison and the Gallows: The Politics of Mass Incarceration in America.* New York: Cambridge University Press.

Gowan, Teresa. 2002. "The Nexus. Homelessness and Incarceration in Two American Cities." *Ethnography* 3:500–534.

Greenberg, Jack. 1994. *Crusaders in the Courts: How a Dedicated Band of Lawyers Fought for the Civil Rights Revolution.* New York: Basic.

Greene, Judith A. 2002. "Entrepreneurial Corrections: Incarceration as Business Opportunity." In *Invisible Punishment: The Collateral Consequences of Mass Imprisonment,* ed. Marc Mauer and Meda Chesney-Lind. New York: New Press.

Greenhouse, Linda. 2000. "Justices Allow Segregation of Inmates with HIV." *New York Times,* January 19, A19–A20.

Griswold, Lewis. 1999. "Sheriff Admits Error in TB Case." *Fresno Bee,* August 27, B1–B2.

Haas, Kenneth C. 1993. "Constitutional Challenges to Compulsory HIV Testing of Prisoners and the Mandatory Segregation of HIV-Positive Prisoners." *Prison Journal* 73:391–432.

Hallet, Michael. 2006. *Private Prisons in America: A Critical Race Perspective.* Champaign: University of Illinois Press.

Haltom, William, and Michael McCann. 2004. *Distorting the Law: Politics, Media, and the Litigation Crisis.* Chicago: University of Chicago Press.

Hammett, Theodore M., Cheryl Roberts, and Sofia Kennedy. 2001. "Health-Related Issues in Prisoner Reentry." *Crime and Delinquency* 47:390–409.

Hammett, Theodore M., R. Widom, J. Epstein, M. Gross, S. Sifre, and T. Enos. 1995. *1994 Update: HIV/AIDS and STDs in Correctional Facilities.*

Washington, DC: U.S. Department of Justice, National Institute of Justice.

Haney, Craig. 1998. "Riding the Punishment Wave: On the Origins of Our Devolving Standards of Decency." *Hastings Women's Law Journal* 9:27–78.

Haney, Craig. 2003. "Mental Health Issues in Long-Term Solitary and 'Supermax' Confinement." *Crime and Delinquency* 49:124–56.

Hans, Valerie P. 2000. *Business on Trial: The Civil Jury and Corporate Responsibility.* New Haven: Yale University Press.

Hart, Nicolette. 1997. "The Social and Economic Environment and Human Health." In *Oxford Textbook of Public Health,* vol. 1, 95–123, ed. Roger Detels, et al. 3d ed. Oxford: Oxford University Press.

Herivel, Tara, and Paul Wright. 2003. *Prison Nation: The Warehousing of America's Poor.* New York: Routledge.

Herman, Susan N. 1998. "Slashing and Burning Prisoners' Rights: Congress and the Supreme Court in Dialogue." *Oregon Law Review* 77:1229–1303.

Hill, Amy. 2002. "Death through Administrative Indifference: The Prison Litigation Reform Act Allows Women to Die in California's Substandard Prison Health Care System." *Hastings Women's Law Journal* 13:223–59.

Hoover, Donald R., Alfred J. Saah, Helena Bacellar, John Phair, Roger Detels, Roger Anderson, and Richard A. Kaslow. 1993. "Clinical Manifestations of AIDS in the Era of Pneumocystis Prophylaxis." *New England Journal of Medicine* 329:1922–26.

Hornblum, Allen. 1999. *Acres of Skin: Human Experiments at Holmesburg Prison.* New York: Routledge.

Horne, Jed. 2006. *Breach of Faith: Hurricane Katrina and the Near Death of a Great American City.* New York: Random House.

Irwin, John. [1970] 1987. *The Felon.* Reprint, Berkeley: University of California Press.

Jackall, Robert. 1988. *Moral Mazes: The World of Corporate Managers.* New York: Oxford University Press.

Jacobs, James. 1977. *Stateville: The Penitentiary in Mass Society.* Chicago: University of Chicago Press.

Jacobs, Leslie. 2007. "Rights and Quarantine During the SARS Global Health Crisis: Differentiated Legal Consciousness in Hong Kong, Shanghai, and Toronto." *Law and Society Review* 41:511–52.

Jacobson, Michael. 2006. *Downsizing Prisons: How to Reduce Crime and End Mass Incarceration.* New York: New York University Press.

Jacobson-Hardy, Michael. 2002. "Behind the Razor Wire: A Photographic Essay." *Ethnography* 3:399–415.

Johnson, Heather Beth. 2006. *The American Dream and the Power of Wealth:*

Choosing Schools and Inheriting Inequality in the Land of Opportunity. New York: Routledge.

Jones, James H. 1993. *Bad Blood: The Tuskegee Syphilis Experiment.* Rev. ed. New York: Free Press.

Jurgens, Ralf. 1994. "Developments in Criminal Law and Criminal Justice: Sentenced to Prison, Sentenced to Death? HIV and AIDS in Prisons." *Criminal Law Forum* 5:763–87.

Kim, Jim Yong, Joyce V. Milen, Alec Irwin, and John Gershman. 2000. *Dying for Growth: Global Inequality and the Health of the Poor.* Monroe, ME: Common Courage Press.

Klinenberg, Eric. 2003. *Heatwave: A Social Autopsy of Disaster in Chicago.* Chicago: University of Chicago Press.

Kral, Alex, Ricky N. Bluthenthal, Robert E. Booth, and John K. Watters. 1998. "HIV Seroprevalence among Street-Recruited Injection Drug and Crack Cocaine Users in 16 U.S. Municipalities." *American Journal of Public Health* 91:108–13.

Kruse, Kevin M. 2005. *White Flight: Atlanta and the Making of Modern Conservatism.* Princeton: Princeton University Press.

Kupers, Terry. 2001. *Prison Madness: The Mental Health Crisis behind Bars and What We Must Do about It.* New York: Jossey-Bass.

La Ganga, Maria L., and Paul Richter. 1996. "Clinton, Dole Deliver Tough Talks on Crime." *San Francisco Chronicle,* September 17, A3–A4.

Levenson, Jacob. 2004. *The Secret Epidemic: The Story of AIDS and Black America.* New York: Pantheon.

Lindblom, Charles E. 1959. "The Science of Muddling Through." *Public Administration Review* 19:79–88.

Lipsitz, George. 1998. *The Possessive Investment in Whiteness: How White People Profit from Identity Politics.* Philadelphia: Temple University Press.

Liptak, Adam. 2003. "Alabama Prison at Center of Suit over AIDS Policy." *New York Times,* October 26, 14–19.

Ludlow, Randy. 2003. "Critical Care." *Columbus Dispatch,* August 24, 1A–3A.

Lynch, Mona. 1998. "Waste Managers? The New Penology, Crime Fighting, and Parole Agent Identity." *Law and Society Review* 32:839–69.

Maddow, Rachel. 2001. "HIV/AIDS and Health Care Reform in British and American Prisons." PhD diss., University of Oxford.

Marable, Manning. 1991. *Race, Reform, and Rebellion: The Second Reconstruction in Black America.* Jackson: University Press of Mississippi.

March, James G., and John P. Olsen. 1979. *Ambiguity and Choice.* Bergen, Norway: Universitetsforlaget.

Marchetti, Anne-Marie. 2002. "Carceral Impoverishment: Class Inequality in the French Penitentiary." *Ethnography* 3:417–34.

Masci, David. 1994. "The Modified Crime Bill." *Congressional Quarterly Weekly,* August 27, 2490–94.

Massey, Douglas S., and Nancy A. Denton. 1993. *American Apartheid: Segregation and the Making of the Underclass.* Cambridge, MA: Harvard University Press.

Massing, Michael. 2000. *The Fix.* Berkeley: University of California Press.

Mauer, Marc, and Meda Chesney-Lind. 2002. *Invisible Punishment: The Collateral Consequences of Mass Imprisonment.* New York: Free Press.

McCann, Michael. 1994. *Rights at Work: Pay Equity Reform and the Politics of Legal Mobilization.* Chicago: University of Chicago Press.

McCorkel, Jill. Forthcoming. *Unruly Subjects: Gender, Punishment, and the Subversion of the Self.* Berkeley: University of California Press.

McDonald, Douglas C. 1995. *Managing Prison Health Care Costs.* Washington, DC: National Institute of Justice.

McDonald, Douglas C. 1999. "Medical Care in Prisons." *Crime and Justice* 26:427–28.

McDonald, Joe. 2007. "Sweeping Sex Scandal Rocks Monroe Prison." *(Allentown) Morning Call,* March 31, A1–A3.

McEwen, Bill. 2005. "Do Graffiti, Eat a Biscuit in Your Pink Underwear." *Fresno Bee,* December 18, B1.

McEwen, Craig A. 1980. "Continuities in the Study of Total and Non-total Institutions." *Annual Review of Sociology* 6:143–85.

McLachlin, Mary, and John Pacenti. 2004. "Jails Medical Provider under Fire." *Palm Beach Post,* February 9, 1A–2A.

Melossi, Dario. 1980. "Punishment and Social Structure." In *Punishment and Penal Discipline,* ed. Tony Platt and Paul Takagi. Berkeley, CA: Crime and Justice Associates.

Michael, Nelson L., and Jerome H. Kim. 1999. *HIV Protocols.* Totowa, NJ: Humana.

Miller, Jerome G. 1991. *Last One over the Wall: The Massachusetts Experiment in Closing Reform Schools.* Columbus: Ohio State University Press.

Moley, Raymond, Jr. 1966. *The American Legion Story.* New York: Duell, Sloan, and Pearce.

Monahan, Susanne C., and Beth A. Quinn. 2006. "Beyond 'Bad Apples' and 'Weak Leaders': Toward a Neo-institutional Explanation of Organizational Deviance." *Theoretical Criminology* 10:361–85.

Mooney, Tom. 1994. "The State Prison May Soon Be Free from Federal Court Supervision for the First Time since 1977." *Providence Journal-Bulletin,* March 19, 1A–3A.

Moore, Solomon. 2007. "New Court to Address California Prison Crowding." *New York Times,* July 24, A16.

Morris, Aldon. 1984. *The Origins of the Civil Rights Movement: Black Communities Organizing for Change.* New York: Macmillan.

Morris, Aldon. 1992. "Political Consciousness and Collective Action." In *The Frontiers of Social Movement Theory,* ed. Aldon Morris and Carol Mueller. New Haven: Yale University Press.

Musheno, Michael C., Peter R. Gregware, and Kriss A. Drass. 1991. "Court Management of AIDS Disputes: A Sociolegal Analysis." *Law and Social Inquiry* 16:737–74.

Nagel, William G. 1973. *The New Red Barn: A Critical Look at the Modern American Prison.* New York: Walker and Company.

Navarro, Vicente. 1984. "Selected Myths Guiding the Reagan Administration's Health Policies." *Journal of Public Health Policy* 5:65–73.

Navarro, Vicente. 1986. *Crisis, Health, and Medicine: A Social Critique.* New York: Tavistock.

Neubeck, Kenneth J., and Noel A. Cazenave. 2001. *Welfare Racism: Playing the Race Card against America's Poor.* New York: Routledge.

Newman, Jon O. 1996. "Pro Se Prisoner Litigation: Looking for Needles in Haystacks." *Brooklyn Law Review* 62:519–27.

New York State Special Commission on Attica. 1972. *Attica: The Official Report of the New York State Commission on Attica.* New York: Praeger.

Nicholson-Crotty, Jill, and Sean Nicholson-Crotty. 2004. "Social Construction and Policy Implementation: Inmate Health as a Public Health Issue." *Social Science Quarterly* 85:240–56.

Nicholson-Crotty, Sean. 2004a. "The Impact of Sentencing Guidelines on State-Level Sanctions: An Analysis over Time." *Crime and Delinquency* 50:395–411.

Nicholson-Crotty, Sean. 2004b. "The Politics and Administration of Privatization: Contracting Out for Corrections Management in the United States." *Policy Studies Journal* 32:41–56.

Oliver, Melvin L., and Thomas Shapiro. 1997. *Black Wealth/White Wealth: A New Perspective on Racial Inequality.* New York: Routledge.

Ortega, Tony. 1999. "109 Degrees of Incarceration." *Phoenix New Times,* May 6, 1–3.

Oshinsky, David M. 1997. *Worse than Slavery: Parchman Farm and the Ordeal of Jim Crow Justice.* New York: Free Press.

Oswald, Mark. 1999. "Former Penitentiary Physician Sues over 1993 Firing." *Santa Fe New Mexican,* July 28, B4.

Paget, Marianne A. 2004. *The Unity of Mistakes: A Phenomenological Interpretation of Medical Work.* Philadelphia: Temple University Press.

Peet, Judy. 2004a. "Barring All Reason." *(Newark) Star Ledger,* December 19, 1–9.

Peet, Judy. 2004b. "N.J.'s Women Inmates Tell Their Own Stories of Abuse." *(Newark) Star Ledger,* May 23, 1–4.

Perrow, Charles, and Mauro F. Guillén. 1990. *The AIDS Disaster: The Failure of Organizations in New York and the Nation.* New Haven: Yale University Press.

Perrucci, Robert, Robert M. Anderson, Dan E. Schendel, and Leon E. Trachtman. 1980. "Whistle-Blowing: Professionals' Resistance to Organizational Authority." *Social Problems* 28:149–64.

Pichardo, Nicholson A. 1997. "New Social Movements: A Critical Review." *Annual Review of Sociology* 23:411–30.

Prendergast, Alan. 1999. "How a Private Prison Brought Jobs—and Violence, Corruption, and Scandal—to Burlington." *Denver Westword,* September 9, 1–11.

Priest, Dana, and Anne Hull. 2007. "Soldiers Face Neglect, Frustration at Army's Top Medical Facility." *Washington Post,* February 18, A1–A5.

Raynou, Garry. 2003. "Audit Rips Management of Inmate Health Care." *Union Leader,* January 16, A8–A10.

Rhodes, Lorna A. 2004. *Total Confinement: Madness and Reason in the Maximum Security Prison.* Berkeley: University of California Press.

Richard, Michel P. 1986. "Goffman Revisited: Relatives vs. Administrators in Nursing Homes." *Qualitative Sociology* 9:321–38.

Robbins, Ira P. 1999. "Managed Health Care in Prisons as Cruel and Unusual Punishment." *Journal of Criminal Law and Criminology* 90:195–237.

Rogers-Dillon, Robin H., and John David Skrentny. 1999. "Administering Success: The Legitimacy Imperative and the Implementation of Welfare Reform." *Social Problems* 46:13–29.

Rose, Peter Isaac, Myron Glazer, and Penina Migdal Glazer. 1977. *Sociology: Inquiring into Society.* San Francisco: Canfield.

Rothman, David. [1980] 2002a. *Conscience and Convenience: The Asylum and Its Alternatives in Progressive America.* Reprint, New York: Aldine Transaction.

Rothman, David. [1971] 2002b. *The Discovery of the Asylum.* Reprint, New York: Aldine Transaction.

Rubenstein, Gwen, and Debbie Mukamal. 2002. "Welfare and Housing: Denial of Benefits of Drug Offenders." In *Invisible Punishment: The Collateral Consequences of Mass Imprisonment.* New York: New Press.

Rusche, George, and Otto Kirchheimer. 1939. *Punishment and Social Structure.* New York: Russell and Russell.

Salmon, J. Warren. 1990. *The Corporate Transformation of Health Care.* New York: Baywood.

Sanger, Mary Bryna. 2003. *The Welfare Marketplace: Privatization and Welfare Reform.* Washington, DC: Brookings Institution Press.

Schlanger, Margo. 2003. "Inmate Litigation." *Harvard Law Review* 116: 1555–1706.

Schlesinger, Mark. 2005. "The Dangers of the Market Panacea." In *Healthy, Wealthy, and Fair: Health Care and the Good Society,* ed. James A. Morone and Lawrence R. Jacobs. New York: Oxford University Press.

Schneider, Cathy Lisa. 1998. "Racism, Drug Policy, and AIDS." *Political Science Quarterly* 113:427–46.

Scott, Alan. 1990. *Ideology and the New Social Movements.* Berkhamsted, England: Red Star Books.

Sen, Amartya. 2003. Foreword to *Pathologies of Power: Health, Human Rights, and the New War on the Poor,* by Paul Farmer. Berkeley: University of California Press.

Sentementes, Gus G. 2007. "Inmate Health System Faulted; State Audit Finds Staffing Shortages, Stalled Drug Treatment Programs." *Baltimore Sun,* March 1, 5B–6B.

Sered, Susan Starr, and Rushika Fernandopulle. 2005. *Uninsured in America: Life and Death in the Land of Opportunity.* Berkeley: University of California Press.

Shamir, Ronen. 2004. "Between Self-Regulation and Alien Tort Claims: On the Contested Concept of Corporate Social Responsibility." *Law and Society Review* 38:635–64.

Shane, Scott. 2007. "Panel on Problems at Walter Reed Issues Strong Rebuke." *New York Times,* April 12, 14–15.

Shay, Jonathan. 1994. *Achilles in Vietnam: Combat Trauma and the Undoing of Character.* New York: Scribner.

Shorey, Aranda. 2003. "Phoenix Sizzling through Hottest July on Record." Associated Press, July 25.

Shurley, Traci, and Nell Smith. 2003. "Report Rips Conditions at Two Arkansas Prisons." *Arkansas Democrat-Gazette,* December 4, 1–2.

Siegal, Nina. 1998. "Lethal Lottery." *POZ,* November, http://www.poz.com/articles/233_1659.shtml.

Sillen, Robert. 2006. "Cruel and Unusual Prison Health Care." *Sacramento Bee,* October 8, E1–E4.

Silverman, Amy. 1996. "Death and Laxness; If the Jailers Had Paid Attention, They Might Have Noticed that Jose Rodriquez Was Dying." *Phoenix New Times,* June 6, 1–8.

Simon, Herbert A. 1976. *Administrative Behavior: A Study of Decision-Making Processes in Administrative Organizations.* 3d ed. New York: Free Press.

Simon, Jonathan. 1997. *Poor Discipline: Parole and the Social Control of the Un-*

derclass, 1890–1990. Paperback ed. Chicago: University of Chicago Press.

Simon, Jonathan. 2007. *Governing through Crime: How the War on Crime Transformed American Democracy and Created a Culture of Fear.* New York: Oxford University Press.

Skolnick, Andrew. 1999. Reply to letters to the editor. *Journal of the American Medical Association* 281:1890–91.

Sloop, John M. 1996. *The Cultural Prison: Discourse, Prisoners, and Punishment.* Tuscaloosa: University of Alabama Press.

Smith, George P. 2000. "Euphemistic Codes and Tell-Tale Hearts: Humane Assistance in End-of-Life Cases." *Case Western Reserve University Health Matrix: Journal of Law-Medicine* 10:175–203.

Smith, Greg. 1999. "Prison System Struggles to Provide Health Care." Associated Press, October 23.

Spade, William. 1996. "Beyond the 100:1 Ratio: Towards a Rational Cocaine Sentencing." *Arizona Law Review* 38:1233–89.

Spelman, William. 2000. "The Limited Importance of Prison Expansion." In *The Crime Drop in America,* ed. Alfred Blumstein and Joel Wallman. New York: Cambridge University Press.

Starr, Paul. 1982. *The Social Transformation of American Medicine.* New York: Basic.

Steiner, Benjamin D. 2001. "The Consciousness of Crime and Punishment: Reflections on Identity Politics and Lawmaking in the War on Drugs." *Studies in Law, Politics, and Society* 23:187–214.

Steiner, Benjamin D., and Victor Argothy. 2001. "White Addiction: Racial Inequality, Racial Ideology, and the War on Drugs." *Temple Political and Civil Rights Review* 10:443–75.

Stockdill, Brett. 2003. *Activism against AIDS: At the Intersections of Sexuality, Race, Gender, and Class.* Boulder, CO: Lynne Rienner.

Stohr, Mark K., Craig Hemmens, Misty Kifer, and Mary Schoeler. 2000. "We Know It, We Just Have to Do It: Perceptions of Ethical Work in Prisons and Jails." *Prison Journal* 80:126–50.

Stoller, Nancy. 1998. *Lessons from the Damned: Queers, Whores, and Junkies Respond to AIDS.* New York: Routledge.

Stoller, Nancy. 2001. "Improving Access to Health Care for California's Women Prisoners." Working paper, California Policy Research Center. http://www.ucop.edu/cprc/documents/stollerpaper.pdf.

Stoller, Nancy. 2003. "Space, Place, and Movement as Aspects of Health Care in Three Women's Prisons." *Social Science and Medicine* 56:2263–75.

Stone, Deborah. 2005. "How Market Ideology Guarantees Racial Inequality." In *Healthy, Wealthy, and Fair: Health Care and the Good Society,* ed.

James A. Morone and Lawrence R. Jacobs. New York: Oxford University Press.

Stucky, Thomas D., Karen Heimer, and Joseph B. Lang. 2007. "A Bigger Piece of the Pie? State Corrections Spending and the Politics of Social Order." *Journal of Research in Crime and Delinquency* 44:91–123.

Sturm, Susan P. 1993. "The Legacy and Future of Corrections Litigation." *University of Pennsylvania Law Review* 142:639–738.

Sward, Susan, and Bill Wallace. 1994. "Health Care Crisis behind Bars: Ailing Inmates Suffer from Lack of Care." *San Francisco Chronicle,* October 3, A1–A11.

Sykes, Gresham. [1958] 1974. *The Society of Captives: A Study in a Maximum Security Prison.* Reprint, Princeton: Princeton University Press.

Tabet, Stephen. 2003. "Expert Report of Stephen Tabet, August 26, 2000." Available at the Web site of the Southern Center for Human Rights, at http://www.schr.org/prisonsjails/news/Limestone/Limestone.html.

Tabet, Stephen. 2004. "Supplemental Report of Stephen Tabet, March 11, 2004." Available at the Web site of the Southern Center for Human Rights, at http://www.schr.org/prisonsjails/news/Limestone/Limestone.html.

Talvi, Silja J. A. 2003. "Hepatitis C." In *Prison Nation: The Warehousing of America's Poor,* ed. Tara Herivel and Paul Wright. New York: Routledge.

Taylor, Judith. 2006. "Who Manages Feminist-Inspired Reform? An In-Depth Look at Title IX Coordinators." In *The New Civil Rights Research: A Constitutive Approach,* ed. Benjamin Fleury-Steiner and Laura-Beth Nielsen. Burlington, VT: Ashgate.

Teeters, Negley. 1955. *The Cradle of the Penitentiary: The Walnut Street Jail at Philadelphia, 1773–1835.* Philadelphia: Pennsylvania Prison Society.

Toch, Hans. 2001. "Future of Supermax Confinement." *Prison Journal* 81:376–88.

Tonry, Michael. 1995. *Malign Neglect: Race, Crime, and Punishment in America.* New York: Oxford University Press.

Treichler, Paula A. 1999. *How to Have Theory in an Epidemic: Cultural Chronicles of AIDS.* Durham, NC: Duke University Press.

Urbina, Ian. 2006. "Panel Suggests Using Inmates in Drug Trials." *New York Times,* August 13, A1.

Vaughan, Diane. 1996. *The Challenger Launch Decision: Risky Technology, Culture, and Deviance at NASA.* Chicago: University of Chicago Press.

Vaughn, Michael S. 1999. "Penal Harm Medicine: State Tort Remedies for Delaying and Denying Health Care to Prisoners." *Crime, Law, and Social Change* 31:273–302.

Vaughn, Michael S., and Leo Carroll. 1998. "Separate and Unequal: Prison versus Free-World Medical Care." *Justice Quarterly* 15:3–40.

Vaughn, Michael S., and Linda G. Smith. 1999. "Practicing Penal Harm Medicine in the United States: Prisoners' Voices from Jail." *Justice Quarterly* 16:175–231.

von Zielbauer, Paul. 2005a. "Harsh Medicine: As Health Care in Jails Goes Private, 10 Days Can Be a Death Sentence." *New York Times,* February 27, A1–A19.

von Zielbauer, Paul. 2005b. "Harsh Medicine: A Company's Troubled Answer for Prisoners with H.I.V." *New York Times,* August 1, A1–A12.

Wagster, Emily. 2001. "Mississippi Opens Education, Drug-Treatment Programs to HIV-Positive Inmates." Associated Press, April 30.

Walzer, Peter D. 2004. *Pneumocystis Carinii Pneumonia.* 2nd ed. New York: Marcel Dekker.

Wacquant, Loïc. 2001a. "Deadly Symbiosis: When Ghetto and Prison Meet and Mesh." *Punishment and Society* 3:95–134.

Wacquant, Loïc. 2001b. "The Penalization of Poverty and the Rise of Neoliberalism." *European Journal of Criminal Policy and Research* 9:401–12.

Wacquant, Loïc. 2002. "The Curious Eclipse of Prison Ethnography in the Age of Mass Incarceration." *Ethnography* 3:372–97.

Ward, Mike, and Bill Bishop. 2001. "Sick in Secret: The Hidden World of Prison Health Care." *Houston Press,* December 16, 1–5.

Warren, Jennifer. 2007. "Sending Prisoners Out of State to Ease Crowded Facilities Is Ruled Illegal." *Los Angeles Times,* February 21, A1–A3.

Watters, John K., and D. K. Lewis. 1990. "HIV Infection, Race, and Drug Treatment History." Letter. *AIDS* 4:697.

Wedge, David. 2001. "Jail Nurse Speaks Out after Oct. MCI Sweep—Calls Prison Life 'Sadistic.'" *Boston Herald,* February 5, 8–10.

Weick, Karl E. 1979. *The Social Psychology of Organizing.* Reading, MA: Addison-Wesley.

Western, Bruce. 2006. *Punishment and Inequality in America.* New York: Russell Sage Foundation.

Western, Bruce, and Katherine Beckett. 1999. "How Unregulated Is the U.S. Labor Market? The Penal System as a Labor Market Institution." *American Journal of Sociology* 104:1030–60.

Western, Bruce, Becky Pettit, and Josh Guetzkow. 2002. "Black Economic Progress in the Era of Mass Incarceration." In *Invisible Punishment: The Collateral Consequences of Mass Imprisonment,* ed. Marc Mauer and Meda Chesney-Lind. New York: New Press.

Whitman, David. 1990. "Inside an AIDS Colony." *U.S. News and World Report,* January 29, 20–26.

Williams, Lee, and Esteban Parra. 2005. "Accountability for Deadly Prisons." *(Wilmington, DE) News Journal,* September 28.

Wilson, Bobby M. 2000. *Race and Place in Birmingham: The Civil Rights and Neighborhood Movements.* Lanham, MD: Rowman and Littlefield.

Wilson, James Q. 1975. *Thinking about Crime.* New York: Basic Books.

Wood, Peter B., and R. Gregory Dunaway. 2003. "Consequences of Truth-in-Sentencing: The Mississippi Case." *Punishment and Society* 5:139–54.

Wood, Phillip J. 2003. "The Rise of the Prison Industrial Complex in the United States." In *Capitalist Punishment: Prison Privatization and Human Rights,* ed. Andrew Coyle, Allison Campbell, and Rodney Neufeld. Atlanta: Clarity.

Wystma, Laura A. 1995. "Punishment for 'Just Us': A Constitutional Analysis of the Crack Cocaine Sentencing Statutes." *George Mason Independent Law Review* 3:473–513.

Yackle, Larry W. 1989. *Reform and Regret: The Story of Federal Judicial Involvement in the Alabama Prison System.* New York: Oxford University Press.

Young, Warren, and Mark Brown. 1993. "Cross-National Comparisons of Imprisonment." In *Crime and Justice: A Review of Research,* vol. 17, ed. Michael Tonry. Chicago: University of Chicago Press.

Zahn, Mary, and Jessica McBride. 2000. "A Wisconsin Prison Term Can Equal a Death Sentence." *Milwaukee Journal Sentinel,* October 22, 1A–13A.

Zimring, Franklin G., and Gordon Hawkins. 1991. *The Scale of Imprisonment.* Chicago: University of Chicago Press.

Zimring, Franklin G., Gordon Hawkins, and Sam Kamin. 2003. *Punishment and Democracy: Three Strikes and You're Out in California.* New York: Oxford University Press.

AUTHOR INDEX

Acton, Andy, 4, 185nn. 9–10
Albertini, William Oliver, Jr., 187n. 15
Albiston, Catherine R., 201n. 28
Alexander, Elizabeth, 41, 192n. 40,
    203n. 25
Altice, Frederick, 27
Anderson, Elijah, 196n. 62
Anderson, Robert M. (Perrucci et al.
    1980), 206n. 8
Anderson, Roger (Hoover et al. 1993),
    188n. 28
Andreas, Peter (Bertram et al. 1996),
    196n. 44
Applegate, Brandon K., 193n. 16
Argothy, Victor, 194n. 28
Arriola, Kimberly Jacob, 198n. 92

Bacellar, Helena (Hoover et al. 1993),
    188n. 28
Barker, Vanessa, 186n. 13
Barry, Ellen, 72, 78, 79, 106, 199n. 1,
    200nn. 20, 22, 27
Bauer, Scott, 210n. 10
Beckett, Katherine, 46, 47, 186n. 13,
    193nn. 14, 23
Belkin, Lisa, 185n. 54
Benjamin, Elizabeth, 196n. 50
Bertram, Eva, 54, 196n. 44
Bidwell, Carol, 198n. 94
Bishop, Bill, 198n. 96, 207nn. 23–24,
    210nn. 2–3 (app. B)
Blachman, Morris J. (Bertram et al.
    1996), 196n. 44
Bluthenthal, Ricky N., 196n. 46
Bonilla-Silva, Eduardo, 209n. 60
Booth, Robert E. (Kral et al. 1998),
    196n. 46

Boreman, Brian D., 195n. 32
Braithwaite, Ronald L., 198n. 92
Brown, Mark, 193n. 19
Brown, T. M., 206n. 47
Brown, Wendy, 47, 192n. 12, 193n. 15
Buckley, William F., 52, 195n. 36
Burawoy, Michael, 13, 187n. 13
Burton, Greg, 210n. 7
Byrd, W. Michael, 12, 50, 162, 163,
    187n. 11, 194nn. 26, 28, 204n. 13,
    209nn. 51, 54–55, 58

Caldicott, Helen, 192n. 7
Calhoun, Craig, 199n. 15
Carroll, Leo, 190n. 16
Cazenave, Noel A., 60, 61, 197n. 68
Chesney-Lind, Meda, 48, 186n. 7,
    193nn. 17–18
Clayton, Linda A., 12, 50, 162, 163,
    187n. 11, 194nn. 26, 28, 204n. 13,
    209nn. 51, 54–55, 58
Clear, Todd R., 33, 48, 190n. 17, 193n.
    16
Clemmer, Donald, 8–9, 11, 186n. 1
Cloud, David S., 189n. 50
Cohen, Cathy J., 52–53, 195n. 38
Cohen, Stanley, 186n. 2
Cole, David, 194n. 27
Comfort, Megan L., 186n. 14, 193n.
    17, 206n. 41
Cook, Rhonda, 192n. 39
Crenshaw, Kimberle, 195n. 34
Crowder, Carla, 14, 98, 99, 114, 115, 122,
    132, 138, 139, 168, 169, 170, 174,
    187nn. 17–18, 202nn. 2–3, 202nn.
    4–5, 7–9, 204nn. 1, 3–4, 8, 11, 12, 16,
    205nn. 19, 29, 206n. 43, 210n. 1 (epi.)

Cullen, Francis T., 193n. 16

Davis, Maia, 63, 197n. 75
Day, Dawn, 55, 196n. 47
Denton, Nancy A., 196n. 62
Detels, Roger (Hoover et al. 1993), 188n. 28
Dimaggio, Paul J., 188n. 40, 202n. 19
Domino, John, 198n. 92
Drass, Kris A., 187n. 14
Dunaway, R. Gregory, 152, 206n. 15, 207n. 17
Dvorak, Richard, 194n. 30, 195n. 35

Edelman, Lauren B., 82, 201n. 28
Eigenberg, Helen, 190n. 15
Enos, Tammy (Hammett et al. 1995), 191n. 34, 208n. 35
Epstein, Edward, 194n. 25
Epstein, Joel (Hammett et al. 1995), 191n. 34, 208n. 35
Erlanger, Howard S., 201n. 28
Ermann, David M., 189n. 41

Farmer, Paul, 160, 161, 196n. 41, 198n. 94, 208nn. 44, 46
Feeley, Malcolm M., 43, 46, 76, 99, 159, 160, 192nn. 1, 12, 199nn. 5, 13–14, 202n. 6, 208nn. 41, 44
Fernandopulle, Rushika, 58, 120, 163, 164, 187n. 9, 191n. 2, 196nn. 59–60, 204nn. 13, 15, 209nn. 56–57
Fisher, Bonnie S., 193n. 16
Fleury-Steiner, Benjamin, 191nn. 36–38, 195n. 34, 199n. 1, 201n. 30
Foucault, Michel, 117, 204n. 9
Friedman, Milton, 43, 44, 192n. 6
Fries, Jacob H., 210n. 5 (app. B)

Garland, David, 46, 161, 162, 186nn. 7, 13, 192n. 11, 209nn. 49–50
Gerber, David, 26, 189nn. 47–48
Gerrit, Jeff, 190n. 10
Gershman, John (Kim et al. 2000), 204n. 13

Gilens, Martin, 197n. 70
Gilman, Sander L., 187n. 15
Glasser, Ira, 193n. 22
Glazer, Myron, 186n. 5
Glazer, Penina Mygdal, 186n. 5
Goffman, Erving, 10, 176, 186n. 6
Goifman, Kiko, 186n. 14
Gostin, Lawrence O., 191n. 21
Gottschalk, Marie, 46, 49, 186n. 13, 192n. 11, 193n. 20, 207n. 16
Gowan, Teresa, 186n. 14
Greenberg, Jack, 199n. 7
Greene, Judith A., 192n. 2
Greenhouse, Linda, 202n. 15
Gregware, Peter R., 187n. 14
Griswold, Lewis, 198n. 4
Gross, Michael (Hammett et al. 1995), 191n. 34, 208n. 35
Guetzkow, Josh, 208n. 43
Guillén, Mauro F., 52, 187n. 14, 195n. 37

Haas, Kenneth C., 202n. 13
Hallet, Michael, 192n. 2
Haltom, William, 197n. 79
Hammett, Theodore M., 27, 38, 191n. 34, 207n. 25, 208n. 35
Haney, Craig, 69, 189n. 55, 198n. 98
Hans, Valerie, 197n. 79
Hart, Nicolette, 194n. 26
Hawkins, Gordon, 186n. 13, 207n. 16
Heimer, Karen, 206n. 13
Hemmens, Craig (Stohr et al. 2000), 190n. 15
Herivel, Tara, 198n. 95
Herman, Susan N., 73, 199n. 3
Hill, Amy, 198n. 86
Hodge, Jessica, 201n. 30
Hoover, Donald, 188n. 28
Hornblum, Allen, 153, 207nn. 20–21
Horne, Jed, 209n. 59
Hull, Anne, 26, 189n. 49

Irwin, Alec (Kim et al. 2000), 204n. 13
Irwin, John, 186n. 2

Oliver, Melvin L., 196n. 2
Olsen, John P., 189n. 40
Ortega, Tony, 199n. 99
Oshinsky, David M., 29, 189n. 1
Oswald, Mark, 206n. 53

Pacenti, John, 206n. 51
Paget, Marianne A., 32, 190n. 12
Parra, Esteban, 208n. 32
Peet, Judy, 206n. 48, 210n. 12
Perrow, Charles, 52, 187n. 14, 195n. 37
Perrucci, Robert, 147, 206n. 8
Pettit, Becky, 208n. 43
Phair, John (Hoover et al. 1993), 188n. 28
Pichardo, Nicholson A., 199n. 15
Powell, Walter W., 188n. 40, 202n. 19
Prendergast, Alan, 210n. 6
Priest, Dana, 26, 189n. 49

Quinn, Beth A., 24, 149, 175, 176, 189nn. 44, 46, 190n. 14, 206n. 10

Raynou, Gary, 210n. 9
Rhodes, Lorna A., 186n. 14
Richard, Michel P., 22, 23, 175, 176, 188nn. 37–39
Richter, Paul, 199n. 100
Robbins, Ira P., 37, 191nn. 30–31
Roberts, Cheryl, 207n. 25
Rogers-Dillon, Robin H., 202n. 19
Rose, Peter Isaac, 186n. 5
Roston, Aram, 4, 185n. 8
Rothman, David, 57, 162, 186n. 2, 196n. 54, 209n. 50
Rubenstein, Gwen, 208n. 43
Rubin, Edward L., 76, 199nn. 5, 13–14
Rusche, George, 8, 46, 171, 186n. 1, 192nn. 9–10, 210n. 5 (epi.)

Saah, Alfred J. (Hoover et al. 1993), 188n. 28
Salmon, J. Warren., 209n. 53
Sanger, Mary Bryna, 61, 192n. 3, 197n. 69

Schendel, Dan E. (Perrucci et al. 1980), 206n. 8
Schlanger, Margo, 65, 66, 67, 74, 197nn. 80–83, 198nn. 84, 97, 199n. 6
Schlesinger, Mark, 36, 191n. 28
Schneider, Cathy Lisa, 55, 196n. 45
Scholer, Mary (Stohr et al. 2000), 190n. 15
Scott, Alan, 76, 199n. 15
Sen, Amartya, 195n. 40
Sentementes, Gus G., 210n. 13
Sered, Susan Starr, 58, 120, 163, 164, 187n. 9, 191n. 2, 196nn. 59–60, 204nn. 13, 15, 209nn. 56–57
Shamir, Ronen, 192n. 8
Shane, Scott, 210n. 4
Shapiro, Thomas, 196n. 62
Sharpe, Kenneth (Bertram et al. 1996), 196n. 44
Shay, Jonathan, 27, 176, 189nn. 47, 51
Shorey, Aranda, 115, 204n. 6
Shurley, Traci, 210n. 4
Siegal, Nina, 189nn. 52–53, 198n. 96
Sifre, Santiago (Hammett et al. 1995), 191n. 34, 208n. 35
Sillen, Robert, 31, 190n. 9, 200n. 21, 207n. 30
Silverman, Amy, 210n. 1 (app. B)
Simon, Herbert A., 189n. 40
Simon, Jonathan, 34, 35, 160, 161, 191nn. 22–24, 208n. 45, 209n. 48
Skolnick, Andrew, 153, 207n. 19
Skrentny, John David, 202n.19
Sloop, John M., 185n. 11, 208n. 33
Smith, George, 135, 205n. 35
Smith, Greg, 201n. 11
Smith, Linda G., 141, 150, 190n. 16, 191n. 25, 206nn. 47, 11 (concl.)
Smith, Nell, 210n. 4
Spade, William, 194n. 29
Starr, Paul, 12, 187n. 10
Steiner, Benjamin, 193n. 21, 194n. 28
Stockdill, Brett, 77, 200n. 18
Stohr, Mark K., 190n. 15
Stoller, Nancy, 32, 33, 80, 81, 117, 119, 130, 138, 150, 190n. 13, 200nn. 19,

25–26, 204nn. 10, 14, 205n. 28, 206n. 41
Stone, Deborah, 54, 196n. 43
Stucky, Thomas D., 206n. 13
Sturm, Susan P., 75, 103, 104, 199nn. 4, 10, 202nn. 11, 16
Sward, Susan, 190nn. 6–7, 208n. 31
Swearingen, Van, 99, 159, 160, 202n. 6, 208nn. 41, 44
Sykes, Gresham, 8, 9, 186n. 2

Tabet, Stephen, 1, 2, 4, 7, 14, 15, 16, 17, 18, 19, 20, 21, 23, 101, 112, 114, 116, 121, 122, 124, 126, 127, 131, 132, 133, 135, 136, 137, 140, 142, 143, 144, 150, 156, 175, 187n. 20, 188nn. 21–23, 26–27, 29, 204nn. 7, 17, 205nn. 18, 21, 22–26, 30, 33–34, 36–38, 206nn. 40, 42, 1–4 (concl.)
Talvi, Silja J A , 208n. 46
Taylor, Judith, 201n. 28
Teeters, Negley, 191n. 20
Toch, Hans, 189n. 55
Tonry, Michael, 193n. 19
Trachtman, Leon E. (Perrucci et al. 1980), 206n. 8
Treichler, Paula A., 187n. 15

Urbina, Ian, 207n. 22

Vaughan, Diane, 23, 175, 188n. 40, 189nn. 42–43
Vaughn, Michael S., 33, 141, 150, 190n. 16, 191n. 25, 206nn. 47, 11 (concl.)
von Zielbauer, Paul, 188n. 31, 190n. 11, 204n. 3, 206nn. 52, 6–7 (concl.), 9 (concl.)

Wacquant, Loïc, 46, 186n. 14, 193n. 13
Wagster, Emily, 202n. 17
Wallace, Bill, 190nn. 6–7, 208n. 31
Walzer, Peter D., 202n. 10
Ward, Mike, 198n. 96, 207nn. 23–24, 210nn. 2–3 (app. B)
Warren, Jennifer, 207n. 18
Watters, John K. (Bluthenthal et al. 1997; Kral et al. 1998; Watters and Lewis 1990), 196n. 46
Wedge, David, 206n. 50
Weick, Karl E., 189n. 40
Western, Bruce, 46, 47, 48, 160, 186n.13, 193nn. 14, 19, 208n. 43
Whitman, David, 2, 3, 4, 185nn. 2–7
Widom, Rebecca (Hammett et al. 1995), 191n. 34, 208n. 35
Williams, Lee, 208n. 32
Wilson, Bobby M., 59, 60, 196nn 64–66
Wilson, James Q., 43
Wood, Peter B., 152, 206n. 15, 207n. 17
Wood, Phillip J., 192n. 5
Wright, Paul, 198n. 95
Wystma, Laura A., 195nn. 33, 35

Yackle, Larry W., 74, 75, 198n. 92, 199nn. 8, 12
Young, Warren, 193n. 19

Zahn, Mary, 151, 187n. 19, 190nn. 3–4, 206n. 12
Zimring, Franklin G., 186n. 13, 207n. 16

SUBJECT INDEX

Abu Ghraib prison: institutional deviance at, 24, 25, 175, 176; scapegoating of "bad apples," 190n. 14. *See also* Institutional deviance, and decoupling of hierarchical structure

ACLU National Prison Project (NPP): litigation in Alabama by, 2, 74, 75, 103, 104, 107, 108, 140, 145, 174; participation in "No Lost Causes," 203n. 25. *See also* HIV+ prisoner rights, and ACLU NPP's early cases; HIV+ prisoner rights, and Judge Johnson's *Newman* decision

AIDS "cocktails," as recent development in treatment for HIV, 118, 119, 122. *See also* Normalization of prisoner deaths; Tabet report

AIDS wasting, and lack of attention to nutrition of prisoners, 20, 80, 90, 122, 135, 138. *See also* Normalization of prisoner deaths; Tabet report, and mortality reviews

Alabama: Department of Corrections (ADOC), 16, 74, 97, 101, 112, 115, 125, 127, 131, 145; Governor's Task Force on Overcrowding in, 56; high taxes for the poor in, 62, 197n. 71; lack of AIDS treatment for the uninsured in, 56, 57, 58; Mobile AIDS Support Services (MASS), 58; unfunded Medicaid program in, 57. *See also* Habitual Offender Felony Act (HOFA), as cause of overcrowding in Alabama's prisons; Habitual Offender Felony Act

(HOFA), and mass incarceration in Alabama; Habitual Offender Felony Act (HOFA), and racial bias; HIV+ prisoner rights, activism; HIV+ prisoner rights, and Judge Johnson's *Newman* decision; HIV+ prisoner rights, litigation; Kilby Prison; *Leatherwood v. Campbell;* Limestone prison; Naphcare, Inc.

Angola prison, 29

Attica prison, 10, 11, 75, 198nn. 92, 94

Avenal State Prison, 31

Bias, Len, 51, 194n. 29

Bureau of Justice Statistics: report on HIV/AIDS rates of infection in U.S. prisons and number of education programs in U.S. prisons, 158; report on HIV-related prisoner deaths, 54, 170; report on state prison expenditures, 196n. 55. *See also* HIV/AIDS, education programs in U.S. prisons; HIV/AIDS, rates of infection in U.S. prisons; Incarceration rates

Captive institutions: Massachusetts juvenile reform schools, 25, 171; mitigating destructiveness as an approach for governing, 25, 27; and "right to rot," 22, 23; as "total institutions," 10, 32, 186n. 5; Walter Reed Army Medical Center, 26, 165, 171. *See also* Institutional deviance; Normalization of prisoner deaths

Catastrophic jails and prisons in the United States: audit of Arkansas's "grossly understaffed" prison medical services, 178; Colorado prison's failure to treat hepatitis C, 178; deaths of New York prisoners in ten New York City jails, 179; deaths of Texas prisoners that "received poor or very poor care," 177, 178; "gross neglect" of prisoners in Utah's Point of the Mountain prison, 179; gross overcrowding in Florida's Pinellas County Jail, 178; Maricopa County's infamous Ward 41, 177; Maryland's "grossly understaffed" penal system, 180; New Hampshire prison as having an "ineffective organizational structure," 179; New Jersey's prison mental health care "as worst I've seen," 180; numerous problems in Nebraska's prison medical care system, 179; segregating of mentally ill prisoners in the Iowa Fort Madison prison "chaotic Cellblock 220," 179–80; as "snapshots" from 1990 to 2007, 177–80

Chandler, Cynthia, 166, 167, 210n. 62

Clean-needle exchange programs, nonexistent in U.S. penal institutions, 208n. 35

Correctional Health Solutions (CHS): physician browbeating HIV+ prisoners with the Bible, 39; quarantine of all chronically ill prisoners, 39. *See also* Fulton County Jail

Correctional Medical Services (CMS): "we offer cost-predictability," 37; and "widespread problem of incompetent doctors," 207n. 19

Corrections officers: power of unions to frustrate reduction of penal populations, 152; subculture of, 190n. 15

Deaths in Custody Reporting Act (DICRA), statistics on HIV-related prisoner deaths, 208n. 34

Dorm 16: drafts and collapsing infrastructure, 16, 115; outdoor pill line, 14, 16, 39, 130, 131, 137, 143, 169; vermin, insects, and spiders inside, 16, 115. *See also* Captive institutions; *Leatherwood v. Campbell;* Normalization of prisoner deaths; Tabet report, background of

Estelle v. Gamble, 72, 73, 199n. 2

Fulton County Jail, 38, 39, 40, 41, 42

Greifinger, Robert, 37, 38

Habitual Offender Felony Act (HOFA): as cause of overcrowding in Alabama's prisons, 56; and mass incarceration in Alabama, 56; and racial bias, 56

Hamilton prison, 2

Harris v. Thigpen, 202n. 14, 206n. 46

Health care crises: in marginalized communities, 35, 36, 48, 57, 58, 59, 120, 163, 204n. 13; rooted in neoliberal economic policies, 12, 162, 163; in U.S. penal institutions, 30, 32, 33, 80, 81, 117, 119, 130, 138, 141, 150, 177, 178, 179, 180, 191n. 25, 200n. 21, 206n. 41. *See also* Hepatitis C; HIV/AIDS; Medical treatment of prisoners; Neoliberalism, "selfcare" as cultural consequence of; U.S. medical care

Hepatitis C, 1, 5, 11, 28, 88, 153, 155, 156, 161, 178, 208n. 46

HIV/AIDS: and Buckley's "AIDS tatoo" proposal, 52; and early years of the epidemic, 118, 119; education programs in U.S. prisons, 158–59; lack of access to treatment for in U.S. prisons, 27; poor blacks at risk of, 54, 55; rates of infection in U.S.

Law and order politics (*continued*)
See *also* Habitual Offender Felony
Act (HOFA); Prison Litigation Reform Act of 1995 (PLRA); Race,
and hysteria after Len Bias's death;
Race, and "infectious black crack
epidemic," Race, and "playing the
crime card"; Race, and "at risk of
infection"; Race, and war on drugs;
Rockefeller sentencing laws
Leatherwood v. Campbell: and fairness
hearing, 111, 112; and Naphcare,
Inc., 97, 98, 99, 100, 101, 106;
Prison Health Services (PHS) takes
over after, 145, 146, 147, 148; and
SCHR's legal strategy, 95–112; settlement and aftermath of, 143, 144,
145, 146, 147. *See also* Limestone
prison, and audit of segregated
HIV/AIDS ward by Jacqueline
Moore and Associates; Southern
Center for Human Rights (SCHR)
Lima Correctional Facility, 30. *See
also* Prima Care, fails to staff the
Ohio Lima Correctional Facility
pharmacy
Limestone prison: and audit of segregated HIV/AIDS ward by Jacqueline Moore and Associates, 18, 112;
and "deadly conditions," 15, 16, 17;
and early media coverage of "AIDS
colony," 2, 3, 4; and HIV/AIDS
Health Care Unit (HCU), 113–42;
and HIV+ prisoner deaths
(1999–2003), 117–40; and Naphcare, Inc., 115–16; and "story of broken health care system," 18, 19, 20,
21; and "story of patient rights," 21,
22, 23; and "thunderdorm," recent
investigative reports of, 14, 15. *See
also* Dorm 16; Normalization of
prisoner deaths

Madison County Jail, 96, 97
Medical treatment of prisoners: and
conflicts with public health, 37, 38;

as "harsh medicine," 31; and institutional failures across the United
States, 23, 24, 30, 31, 32; and mental
illness, 28; as "penal harm," 33, 48;
proposals to reform, 151, 152, 153,
154, 155, 156, 157; as treating "depersonalized units," 32, 33. *See also*
HIV+ prisoner rights; Normalization of prisoner deaths
Menard prison, 8
Methodology: and "extended case
method," 13, 187n. 13; and "a fuller
account of methods," app. A
Military industrial complex, 44, 192n.
7

Naphcare, Inc., ADOC hires, 99,
100, 115, 116, 117. *See also* Limestone
prison, and Naphcare, Inc.; Normalization of prisoner deaths
NASA shuttle disaster, institutional
deviance at root of, 23, 24. *See also*
Institutional deviance
Neoliberalism: aggressive privatization as imperative of, 44, 45, 46, 47,
48; and *Capitalism and Freedom,* 43,
44; and "corporate social responsibility," 192n. 8; and lack of government intervention in U.S. health
care crisis, 192n. 4; and "neoliberal
penality," 46; and prisons as labor
market institutions, 47; "self-care"
as cultural consequence of, 47, 48.
See also Law and order politics, cost
cutting as by-product of; Privatization
New York State Special Commission
on Attica, and findings of prison
health care failures, 10, 11
Normalization of prisoner deaths:
and "creating alternative spaces of
care," 138, 139, 140, 206n. 41; and
"do not resuscitate," 134–38; and
manifestations of lethal discipline,
121–42; medication adherence
agreement as evidence of, 128; and

Race (*continued*)
54–55; and war on drugs, 51. *See also* Law and order politics, driven by racialized hysteria; Law and order politics, and "southern strategy"
Rockefeller sentencing laws, 56
Shumate v. Wilson, 79, 80, 107, 200n. 23, 202n. 20
Southern Center for Human Rights (SCHR), chap. 5. See also *Leatherwood v. Campbell*
Staph infection: as consequence of untreated HIV, 16, 98, 178; and "plague of boils," 97
Stateville prison, 9, 10

Tabet report: background of, 1, 2, 4, 7, 14, 15, 16, 17, 18, 19, 20, 21, 23, 101, 112, 114, 116; and mortality reviews, 121, 122, 124, 126, 127, 131, 132, 133, 135, 136, 137, 140, 142, 143, 144, 150, 156, 175, 187n. 20. *See also* AIDS "cocktails"; AIDS wasting; Dorm 16; *Leatherwood v. Campbell;* Limestone prison, and "story of broken health care system"; Normaliza-

tion of prisoner deaths; Prisoner deaths, inside Alabama prisons
Tuberculosis (TB): education programs in U.S. prisons, 158, 159; rates of infection in U.S. prisons, 158

U.S. medical care: experiences of the uninsured, 58, 120, 163, 164, 204n. 13; as a "medical industrial complex," 162, 163, 209n. 53; racial inequalities and lack of, 36; as "zero sum medical practice," 12. *See also* Neoliberalism, aggressive privatization as imperative of; Neoliberalism, and "corporate social responsibility"; Neoliberalism, and lack of government intervention in U.S. health care crisis

Walker, Jackie, 109, 110, 203nn. 24–25, 204n. 26
Walnut Street Jail, 34
Walter Reed Army Medical Center, catastrophic conditions of "Building 18," 26, 165, 171
Welfare racism, social, political, and economic functions of, 60, 61